*My dream is that every woman,
everywhere, will know the joy of a
truly safe, comfortable, and
satisfying birthing for herself
and her baby.*

*Marie F. Mongan, 1998*

*HypnoBirthing®* - A Celebration of Life
by Marie F. Mongan, M.Ed., M.Hy.

NOTE: The HypnoBirthing method and this book describing its techniques are not intended to represent a medically and anatomically precise overview of pregnancy and birthing, nor are they designed to represent medical advice or a prescription for medical procedure. The content of this book is not intended to replace the advice of a medical doctor. It is advisable for any pregnant woman to seek the advice of a medical doctor or health care provider before undertaking any pregnancy or labor-related program.

Persons following any course of action recommended in this book or in the HypnoBirthing Program do so of their own free will. Neither the author nor the publisher assumes responsibility for any possible complication related to either the pregnancy or the labor of the participant.

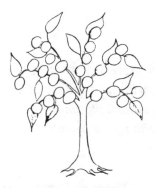

# RIVERTREE PUBLISHING

ISBN 0-9663517-1-1                    Copyright © 1992, 1998, Concord, N.H.

HypnoBirthing is a reserved trade name.          Illustrations: Sheryl Chatterton & R. Heston
Cover design: Ron Leland     Logo: Mary Ann Murphy      Editor: Lisa Smith
HypnoBirthing Institute, P. O. Box 810, Epsom, NH 03234 (603) 798-3286
e-mail: hypnobirthing@hypnobirthing.com                    Website: www.hypnobirthing.com

# *HypnoBirthing*®

# A Celebration of Life

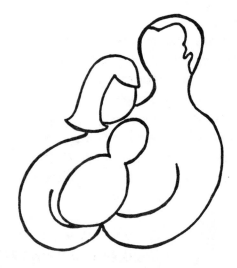

A definitive guide for a safer, easier, more comfortable
birthing in the way that most mirrors nature

Expanded Edition

Marie F. Mongan, M.Ed., M.Hy.

*"It is not only that we want to bring about an easy labor, without risk of injury to the mother or the child; we must go further. We must understand that childbirth is fundamentally a spiritual, as well as a physical, achievement . . . it must be understood that the birth of a child is the ultimate perfection of human love. . . ."*

Dr. Grantly Dick-Read
<u>Childbirth Without Fear</u>, 1953

*From Marcelene Dyer:*

My first child's birth was free of all sensations. I never felt the waves of energy--some call pain.

I know about HypnoBirthing. I came here with this knowledge. Yet, it is only lately that there is this realization.

Somewhere in my innocence, I saw birth as a most spiritual event. I did not buy into the group mentality which links birth with suffering. What I saw was an exhilaration of spirit in meeting this new being who was to share a most sacred journey with me.

My only true goal was to become a mother. I chose not to suffer; yet I did not ask this of God. Instead, I confirmed with Him my ability to give birth to my body's child with a wide-awake wonder. This was granted. I was wide awake. All else was a gift--truly.

Did I "program" my mind during the hours nightly that I knelt in prayer? I used visualization, with my own precious mental pictures of my perfect birth. After months of this ritual, and five weeks before his due date, I saw the birth in a dream. The next night Shane was born, as pictured. I cannot explain all of it. In fact, I still haven't grown into the experience.

I went on to have six more children, five daughters and another son. All births were like the first; I never suffered.

My own book on childbirth is my personal journey of seven births. . . non medical--real, and my commitment to every woman that she can do the same. She only has to get out of her own way.

Marcelene Dyer
Co-author with husband, Wayne Dyer
A Promise Is A Promise

## From Marie F. Mongan, founder of HypnoBirthing:

I'm pleased that your interest in a birthing experience that will be both satisfying and safe for you and your baby has caused you to pick up this book. The HypnoBirthing Method of childbirth is the ideal choice for anyone who shares a concern for the safety and comfort of birthing mothers and their babies.

As yet there is no labor drug proven to be totally safe. In spite of the fact that the drugs most commonly administered in labor have been used for years, data is just now beginning to be gathered; conclusions are yet to come. The HypnoBirthing Method has been developed to teach you self-hypnosis techniques and special ways of working with your body to achieve the satisfying birthing that you seek--free of harmful narcotics and free of the fear that causes pain and discomfort.

This book is the textbook used by clients in HypnoBirthing classes. It outlines the philosophy and many of the techniques that are used by HypnoBirthing mothers. The book, however, is just that--an outline. While you will gain much information from it, it cannot replace the comprehensive instruction that you will receive from attending authorized HypnoBirthing classes. Specific methods for alleviating pain and bringing about a shorter, easier and more comfortable birthing cannot be gleaned from simply reading the book or working with a therapist who is not certified to teach HypnoBirthing techniques.

HypnoBirthing classes are taught in four or five sessions, usually to no more than four to five couples. The number is intentionally kept small to assure individual attention to your needs.

For information on HypnoBirthing classes in your area or information on becoming a Certified HypnoBirthing Practitioner, please contact:

*HypnoBirthing Institute* • P. O. Box 810 • Epsom, N.H. 03234

(603) 798-3286    e-mail: hypnobirthing@hypnobirthing.com    Website: www.hypnobirthing.com

# Table of Contents

# *Dedications*

To my daughter Maura, whose decision to have a child gave me the inspiration to recreate the program of natural birthing through which she was born in 1959--a program that has been waiting these many years to come into being. I salute her choice with loving gratitude.

Marie F. Mongan, 1989

To our four HypnoBirthing grandbabies who were born since the inception of the program: Kyle Patrick, born January 3, 1990; Patrick John, born September 11, 1992; Meghan Taylor, born September 28, 1996; and Melissa Kelley, born November 25, 1996.

To my husband Gene, whom I can't thank enough. He was my patient birthing companion and champion throughout the labor of this expanded edition. Without his love and support, this book would not have been birthed.

Marie F. Mongan, 1998

*"Children are life's most precious resource. They determine our future. They carry on family legacies. They inspire our everyday lives and provide us with an opportunity to make a difference."*

*Jan Blaustone*
*The Joy of Parenthood*

# *Appreciation*

It is with gratitude and deep appreciation that I acknowledge:

The late Dr. Grantly Dick-Read, 1890 - 1959, a husband and father, a philosopher, an Englishman, who through his work in obstetrics and his book, *Childbirth Without Fear*, returned to women the gift of their right to truly natural childbirth. He is a prophet whose time is yet to come. His philosophy and work is the basis and the inspiration for this program.

Those several couples who had complete belief in this program and who were willing to place their faith in the HypnoBirthing philosophy, confident that this most natural birthing method would provide for them the fulfillment they were seeking as they experienced the greatest celebration of life--childbirth.

Mary Ann Murphy, dear friend, who put the natural simplicity of the HypnoBirthing philosophy into form in her creation of our logo depicting the love and bonding that takes place during HypnoBirthing.

George Ferren, my right arm, without whom much of this expanded edition would still be in shorthand notes. George kept me on track by producing finished copy almost as fast as I could create drafts.

# The Story Begins

It was June of 1954; I was 21 years old and was sure that the world was mine for the taking. On the 5th of June, I was graduated from a small teachers college in Plymouth, New Hampshire. I had already signed a contract to teach in the fall; and now, with degree in hand, I was realizing the fruition of a childhood dream. I was going to be a teacher.

One week later, on the 12th, I was married. It was a fairytale wedding between high school sweethearts. Because my husband was in the service and his unit was put on alert just three days before our marriage, we had only a brief weekend together after the wedding. He was assigned to overseas duty for four months.

I began teaching in September and knew that I had found the niche that would be mine for the rest of my life. My husband was discharged from the service late that fall, and we began our lives together in a small lumber town in the foothills of New Hampshire's White Mountains.

In January I missed a period. I knew it was the result of the bronchitis that attacked me in December and was lingering in full force. A local doctor confirmed my diagnosis. During February and March, the bronchitis was still doing its thing. Unhappy with the treatment that I was receiving and anxious to get my system back on schedule, I decided to make an appointment with my family doctor in my hometown. When we sat in his office after my examination, his diagnosis sent me into a state of shock. I was pregnant.

It had never occurred to us that we were going to have a baby. Neither of us had even considered having a child at that point in our lives. My husband had enrolled in college under the G.I. Bill; I was very involved in lesson plans and adjusting to all of the experiences that come with being a first-year teacher; our marriage was so new; we hadn't even finished furnishing the small, one-bedroom apartment that we were renting; I wasn't sick in the morning; I didn't show any signs of bloating; and my appetite hadn't taken on any bizarre twists. We just couldn't be having a baby now.

For several days I was tempted to go back to the other doctor so he could tell me that it was simply my bronchitis that was raising havoc with my body and I really wasn't going to have a baby.

Then one morning I awakened feeling a strange, exciting glow about myself. There was a voice from deep inside me that kept repeating, "I'm going to have a baby." I felt an exhilaration that was different from anything I have ever felt before, and I liked it. I don't know where it came from; but I do know that from that moment on, I became enthralled with the wonderment of what was happening inside me. I became all consumed with my pregnancy and with thoughts of our new baby. This was not going to be a "usual pregnancy" with aching back, swollen feet, or any of the other complaints that are common to pregnancy; and my birthing was not going to be one of drugged compliance with no recollection of the experience.

The premise that birthing, by nature, had to be a painful ordeal was totally unacceptable to me. I could not believe that a God who had created the body with such perfection could have designed a system of procreation that was flawed. Even more importantly, I could not believe that a loving God would commit so cruel a hoax as to make us sexual beings so that we could conceive and then make the means through which we would birth our children so excruciatingly painful.

I read everything I could get my hands on, and that's when I discovered Dr. Grantly Dick-Read, the father of Natural Childbirth. I knew immediately that his method was the answer to the drug-free, painless birthing that I was seeking. I discarded most of the other negative literature devoted to descriptions of laboring mothers trying to cope with and survive the "excruciating pain of childbirth" and began to focus on Dick-Read's techniques for eliminating the "Fear-Tension-Pain Syndrome." I was excited at having found the Dick-Read method and looked forward to my Natural Childbirth, awake, alert, and free of pain.

I was prepared for natural birthing but was not prepared for the reaction of other people from both within and outside of the medical field. No one thought I was serious about having a baby without having anesthesia. Friends laughed at me for even suggesting that it was possible. Luckily, my husband and my family, accustomed to my propensity for doing the unusual, provided skeptical support.

When it came time for my birthing, I was ridiculed and insulted by anesthesiologists, who were at that time introducing the "caudal," a spinal block. While I was in labor, the nurses kindly reassured me, "When the pains get unbearable, you can have a shot of Demorol to ease them." I was mocked when I refused. Left alone in a dark labor room, listening to the insufferable ticking of a "Baby Ben" clock that was placed by my side so that I could "time" my "labor pains," I found myself ignored by nurses, who wouldn't accept my word for what was happening in my labor. When I insisted that I was ready to push, they told me that when I was ready, I would be, ". . . yelling and screaming like the rest of them." Once in the delivery room, my wrists were strapped to the sides of the delivery table with leather straps; and my legs were tied into the stirrups that held my knees and legs four feet into the air. My head was held as the ether cone was forced onto my face. That was the last I remembered. I awakened sometime later, violently ill from the ether, and was informed that I had "delivered" a beautiful baby boy, whom I would be able to see in the morning. The nurse cautioned me not to be alarmed at the red bruises on his face from the forceps. My husband was allowed to visit me for ten minutes. Neither of us held our son Wayne that evening.

When I saw my baby for the first time, I was horrified to think of what he must have experienced as he was being "yanked" into the world. This certainly was not the natural birthing I had planned. My husband saw our son only through the window of the nursery for the next six days, as no one was allowed to visit when, "The babies are on the floor."

Two years later when I was in labor with our second son Brian, the course of the first stage of labor was as peaceful and comfortable as it had been with my first child; but, again, his birthing was a total blank. When I was finally allowed to see him at the allotted time, I found that again, there were the red blotches on my baby's face from the pressure of forceps. Six days later when Brian and I were discharged from the hospital, my husband was able to hold him for the first time.

Finally in 1959, in my third attempt, I announced to my doctor that I would have the natural birth that I wanted, even if it meant that I would have to travel elsewhere to find a doctor who would listen to my needs as a birthing mother. This included having my husband present in the labor room and in the "delivery" room as our baby was born. To understand how outlandish this request was, you have to realize that in the late 50s husbands were not allowed beyond the lobby of the hospital. There were no lounge areas located near the maternity ward for fathers to pace.

I was successful in obtaining my doctor's support and his promise to give official orders that I was to be accommodated in fulfilling what I believe was the original birth plan. My husband was by my side throughout my 2 1/2 hour labor, and he accompanied me to the "delivery room" and stood by my side while our daughter was born--a first for that hospital and for the entire region. My arms and legs were free; I was wide awake. As before, I had taken no drugs or anesthetics; and my joy was unparalleled. I finally had my fully natural birth. I stood at the nursery window watching them bathe my daughter within minutes of my return to my room--this at a time when women were hardly allowed out of bed for at least a day or more after birthing. "Confinement" at that time was at least five days--six days if a male child had to be circumcised.

Everyone who was with me that evening was on a natural high. My doctor was excited to the extent that he stayed up until three in the morning reading everything he had available on Dr. Grantly Dick-Read's Natural Childbirth. I was told that my birthing was the talk of the entire hospital for three shifts. Unfortunately, this fascination and curiosity on the part of the medical staff was short lived. My birthing was dismissed as a "fluke". I was told that some women have an incredible tolerance to pain, and my baby girl ". . . was only 6lbs. 3ozs." The trail I thought I had blazed was quickly swept over. Nothing changed.

My fourth birthing followed the same smooth path, even though our son Shawn was two pounds heavier than Maura. My doctor, still fascinated, but not at all convinced, told me that he was unbelievably impressed that someone could endure that much pain so calmly and without anesthesia. In spite of my frequent boasts of feeling nothing but tightening sensations, I was not successful in opening his mind to what natural birthing could be for the mothers who were to come after me.

So there we were. Leather straps, ether cones, spinals, and stirrups were to prevail for a long time to come.

Through the years, I shuddered each time I heard a woman speak of having experienced horrific agony in having her baby. It saddened me because I knew that the pain that she felt could have been eased, and in many instances, even eliminated. I felt so helpless. Whenever I spoke of easier childbirth, my listeners looked at me with shock or polite disbelief.

In 1988 I added hypnotherapy to a counseling practice that I had maintained throughout the years when I was dean at a women's college and later in my role as the director of a school of business. Being involved in hypnotherapy caused me to think back to my birthings. I realized for the first time that I had, indeed, used self-hypnosis to achieve the degree of relaxation that made it possible for me to experience painless childbirth. (Grantly Dick-Read emphatically denied that his method is at all connected with hypnosis. He felt that hypnosis brings women to a totally disassociated state that robs them of the beauty of experiencing birthing. We now know that a person who is in a hypnotic state is fully awake and in an even heightened state of awareness.) I was, indeed, in self-hypnosis when I labored with my children.

Not long after I became a hypnotherapist, my daughter Maura told me of her desire to have a child. I was determined that she experience only the very best and most satisfying birthing possible. The thought of developing a birthing program utilizing these techniques was never far from the surface of my mind, and I felt that my being a hypnotherapist would give the program the legitimacy that was lacking before. From this newly awakened interest in birthing came HypnoBirthing. I started making notes in 1989. I delighted in the prospect of developing the program that would allow Maura, who was the first baby in the area to be born with a method of self-hypnosis, to bring her own child into the world with HypnoBirthing. There were two other women preparing for their birthings at the same time, and I prayed that she be the first to birth. She was.

On January 3, 1990, the first HypnoBirthing baby, our grandson Kyle, was born. We had gone full circle--from Maura, the first natural birth baby in the region, to Kyle, the first HypnoBirthing baby. I can't even begin to express how spiritually exciting this was for me.

Maura did not have the benefit of videos or success stories of other women who had birthed their babies through HypnoBirthing. I believe that, on a deeper level, her own birth left an imprint in her subconscious of what birth should be. She fully trusted her body, and it worked for her.

Since then, hundreds more have joined the ranks of HypnoBirthing babies. Because of HypnoBirthing, couples today can look forward to a beautiful, calm and serene birthing experience, where mother, baby and birthing companion combine in joyful bonding.

HypnoBirthing has returned to women their right to call upon their natural birthing instincts, creating one of the most memorable experiences of their lives.

Dr. Christiane Northrup, author of <u>Women's Bodies, Women's Wisdom</u>, expresses it well in her book when she forwards a challenge to all birthing mothers:

"Imagine what might happen if the majority of women emerged from their labor beds with a renewed sense of the strength and power of their bodies, and of their capacity for ecstasy through giving birth. When enough women realize that birth is a time of great opportunity to get in touch with their true power, and when they are willing to assume responsibility for this, we will reclaim the power of birth and help move technology where it belongs--in the service of birthing women, not as their master."

*"If we are to heal the planet, we must begin by healing birthing."*
*Agnes Sallet von Tannenberg*

# The Philosophy
## of
## HypnoBirthing

The HypnoBirthing method of childbirth education is as much a philosophy as it is a technique. It is a rewarding, relaxing, and stress-free method of birthing that teaches a mother, along with her birthing companion, the art and joy of experiencing birth in an easier, more comfortable, and often pain-free manner that most nearly mirrors nature. The HypnoBirthing Program was developed in 1989 by Marie Mongan and is based on the work of English obstetrician, Dr. Grantly Dick-Read, the father of Natural Childbirth. HypnoBirthing proponents subscribe to the belief that when a woman is given the proper preparation for childbirth, she and her birthing companion can experience a safe, serene, and satisfying birthing, free of the fear that causes tension and pain. When mind and body are in harmony, nature is free to function in the same well-designed manner that it does with all other creatures.

The concept of easier birthing is easily understood when you examine the "Robot Theory," based on the belief that only the mind can think. What is experienced in the body is determined in the mind; therefore, what the mind chooses to accept or perceive as being real, the robot body, accordingly, responds to. An example of this control by the mind over the body is the football player who sprains an ankle at the beginning of the last quarter of the game. Because his conscious attention is totally focused on playing that game and winning, he may feel the pressure of the swelling of the ankle but feels no pain. His mind has narrowed its focus and is accepting only the suggestion that he must remain in the game and play his hardest. The pressure of the ankle is relayed by the subconscious mind as only a minor consideration that does not warrant a sympathetic or pain stimuli response. His ankle does not accept the sharp twist as a source of pain because only the mind is able to think or to react to pain stimuli. If there is no pain stimuli, he feels no pain. It is not until the game is over that his mind is again redirected, the message of the sprain is relayed to the mind, and he begins to feel the discomfort.

So, too, in birthing, when the mind accepts the belief that without complication, birthing proceeds naturally, no pain exists, and no pain is experienced. The body's physiological response is to feel only the tightening or pressure of a uterine wave as it goes about its task of dilating the cervix and expelling the baby naturally.

How does the pregnant mind and body learn this belief? By reading and attending childbirth education programs. However, all childbirth education programs are not created equal.

Perhaps the most familiar name in childbirth education is Lamaze. For almost two decades, the well-publicized Lamaze Method was synonymous with Natural Childbirth. The concept of Natural Childbirth, with all of its merits, however, was missing something. Offered to women during the latter part of the third trimester, when their pregnancy was quite advanced, it did little to explore factors other than the physiological aspects of birthing. It failed to consider the impact of a woman's emotional state on her pregnancy and her labor. As the program became diluted over the years, many of the teachers of Lamaze relinquished the name and the concept of Natural Childbirth and surrendered to the rapidly emerging "prepared childbirth" programs. Each of these programs has put its own spin on what prepared childbirth should be, and now there are almost as many differing philosophies as there are classes.

Today, many programs have become information channels for the local hospitals, designed primarily to acquaint you with the "medical model" and educate you to the drugs, technological equipment, and medical procedures that are routinely in use at the hospitals. Some programs teach methods that attempt to take your focus away from the pain so that you will not be so aware of it, training you to cope with pain rather than reduce it or eliminate it. Others suggest that you look upon the pain as an empowerment of your womanhood, something to rise above and triumph over. You are taught to accept the pain of labor as inevitable but not insurmountable. Some teach that you view pain as an unavoidable, but useful, friend that can be tolerated, worked with, and learned from. These techniques are premised on a basic belief that pain must be associated with labor and the pain must somehow be accommodated.

The HypnoBirthing philosophy differs vastly from all of these views. HypnoBirthing is predicated on the belief that as a woman, you can experience birth through your own natural birthing instincts--serenely, comfortably, with dignity, and with as little medical intervention as possible. The program teaches you to go with the natural flow and rhythm of your laboring body; to release your birthing over to your mind and body;

and to trust your body to function as it was intended to, thereby alleviating pain. HypnoBirthing teaches you and your birthing companion to work with natural relaxation techniques so that your body can work with complete neuromuscular harmony, assisting rather than resisting.

HypnoBirthing is a collaborative method of childbirth, not an alternative method. The HypnoBirthing philosophy does not preclude the introduction of medical intervention, per se; it precludes the introduction of arbitrary or unnecessary medical intervention, proposed only for the expediency of "getting 'things' over with." There is no room for this kind of "assembly-line mentality" in today's birthing places. Many birthing places are "suiting up" with soft, gentle colors, and family-oriented ambiance; but there must be a corresponding shift in the birthing philosophy of those who come into these settings to attend mothers in labor. Otherwise, the decor becomes merely a disguise. The emotional and spiritual needs of laboring women and their babies need to be addressed with gentility, patience and kindness.

In addition to teaching techniques for instant relaxation, the program provides fear-release sessions that help you identify and eliminate issues, fears, or negative feelings you may have surrounding your birthing or parenting. When you are free of stress and fear, your body is free of pain-causing tension.

When you have your baby using the HypnoBirthing method, you will not be in a trance or a sleep state. What you will experience is similar to the daydreaming or focusing that occurs when you are engrossed in a book or staring at a fire--when you lose track of what's going on around you. Though you will be totally relaxed, you will also be fully in control. During your birthing you will be aware and even sense your uterine surges, but you will experience them in total harmony of mind and body. You will be very much in charge and can interrupt the relaxed state or resume it at any time you wish to do so.

Through classes taught by professional hypnotherapists, nurses, midwives, and birthing educators, trained in the techniques of hypnoanesthesia, you will become skilled in using your own natural abilities to bring your mind and body into perfect harmony. You will gain an understanding of the physiology of labor that goes beyond what is usually taught in other classes. You will learn special relaxation conditioning and labor techniques that will enable you to connect with and work with your body as you experience labor.

The value of self-hypnosis comes from your learning to reach that level of mind where suggestions that you give yourself effectively influence your physiological experience. Your HypnoBirthing Practitioner will help you learn to reach this level, where you dispel fear, tension, and discomfort during birthing. You will see, hear, and practice these techniques in class and will be given practice tapes to work with at home. When it's time for your baby to be born, you will be awake and involved.

The profound relaxation that you learn will prove to be a valuable skill that can be useful to you throughout your life, not just as you prepare for the birthing of your child. Many couples find that the weeks of preparation in relaxation also have a calming effect upon the baby.

*"Birth savvy mothers who value totally unmedicated and intervention-free birthing, have a new term for it- - 'Pure Birth'."*

*Sears & Sears*
*The Birth Book*

# *A Message to You*

## TO THE MOTHER TO BE

Taking part in the birthing of a child is probably one of the most beautiful times and experiences that you will ever know. Your choosing HypnoBirthing as your birthing method will make the event all the more wonderful and fulfilling.

The realization that you are carrying and will soon give birth to a new life is bound to evoke a number of feelings and emotions that you have never felt before. Like most parents-to-be, much of your thinking is given over to this little baby whom you are carrying and for whose birth you are preparing. This is very important. It is also important to reflect on how very special you are and how special your feelings are about the changes that are taking place in your body and in your life. Naturally, you want to be in control of the entire experience. What you are experiencing is unique to you. You are unique. No matter how many children you have, this particular child will never be physically born again. Its birth can never be duplicated; and there is not another human being in the whole world other than you who could conceive, carry, bond with, and bring this tiny person into the world. This is a once-in-a-lifetime event, and it's only natural that you and your birthing companion are seeking as safe, satisfying, and fulfilling a birthing as is possible.

Your HypnoBirthing classes are designed to enhance those feelings of uniqueness and awe, helping you to reach an awareness of your body as the most perfected instrument of nature--the vehicle through which and from which your child will miraculously develop and enter into this world. Birthing is Nature characterized at its best. It is the implementation of the highest power of life that ensures the survival of the human race. All other works of nature pale by comparison to the miracle of birth, and you are at the heart of that wonderful miracle.

Through HypnoBirthing you will learn how Nature has been working with you from the very beginning of your pregnancy to prepare your body for this great wonder. You will also learn how the body continues to work with you throughout your birthing.

You will come to understand that when you are free of fear and tension, pain is incongruous with the way in which your body was designed to complete its role. With these understandings, you will learn techniques that will allow you to make the entire experience one that will be filled with relaxed expectation and confidence.

## BIRTHING COMPANION

You who are looking forward to serving as a Birthing Companion--husband, partner, friend, sister, mother--have a very special part to play when participating in HypnoBirthing. Countless women who have given birth through this program have laid the success of their birthing experience directly upon the support and assistance of the birth companion. Anyone who observes a HypnoBirthing will bear this out. The support and bonding that take place throughout labor and birthing create a partnership, the beauty of which cannot adequately be described.

The importance of your role as you attend classes, learn techniques to assist the mother during birthing, and help her practice relaxation and visualization can't be overstated. Your willingness to take the lead is a key factor in assuring that the birthing you both have planned becomes a reality, and it will build your partner's confidence. As an integral part of the process, you bring the necessary elements of trust and assurance to the birthing environment. You will be the facilitator--helping her condition her mind to relax in response to your prompts. The attention, understanding, encouragement, comfort, and closeness that you provide create a sharing that is unequaled and help create a bond that will linger throughout your lives.

The sound of your voice and the touch of your hand as you guide the laboring mother through all of the stages of labor provide the basic ingredients to successful HypnoBirthing--a confident, secure, and comfortable mother, who is relaxed and in control.

As a birth companion, you may at first feel unsure about your role in the birthing. This, too, is natural. As you guide the mother during birthing, however, you will quickly sense the importance of your prompts in helping her to maintain the peace and calm that surround the birth.

If you have fear surrounding your ability to watch someone you love experience discomfort, the HypnoBirthing classes will allay those fears. You will come to know that through this program you and the birthing mother will learn techniques that will alleviate the discomfort and possibly even eliminate it. It's your support and love that makes this happen.

Working with her through each uterine surge, you will become fully consumed in her responsiveness, and any awareness of others will totally dissipate. You will instinctively know what you must do, and you will become oblivious to the coming and going of medical caregivers. A woman in labor is vulnerable, sensitive, and usually unassertive. It is you who will be her advocate, her spokesperson, her guide. You will be the liaison between her and the medical staff. Your involvement in preparing the birthing plan and seeing that it is carried out will be one of your most important tasks. Your presence and support, especially during the actual birthing, cannot be equaled; and at the moment of birth, you will feel the exhilaration that comes with knowing that together you have made this miracle one that neither of you will ever forget.

*"If you love the mother and baby, you will care for them as only a loved one can."*
*Penny Simkin*
*The Birth Partner*

# Getting Started

Much of what is written here centers around preparation for birthing your baby at a hospital or birthing center. The fact that there is little mention of home birthing should not be construed as an indication that the HypnoBirthing philosophy precludes home birth. Just the opposite is true. HypnoBirthing is an especially appropriate birthing method for you if you plan to have your baby at home. Very little time or space is devoted to the discussion of home birth because it's presumed that if you have chosen to have your baby in the comfort of your own home with a midwife for your caregiver, you have already determined that you want to have your baby in the most natural setting and with as little intervention as possible. Many midwives, unable and unwilling to introduce artificial drugs and procedures to the birth scene, are adopting the HypnoBirthing philosophy because it adds an even greater dimension to Natural Childbirth--a shorter, easier, serene, and more comfortable labor and birth. Except for references that specifically speak of hospital equipment, procedures, or policies, the information here is applicable to a home birth, a hospital birth, or a birthing center birth.

Whether you birth at home or in a hospital, the term "Natural Childbirth" should not lull you into feeling that HypnoBirthing techniques will come naturally. Perhaps the day will come when we abandon the concept of fear and pain in birthing, and much of what is written here will be obsolete. All birthings will be approached with confidence. I pray that I will soon see the day when mothers will anticipate birthing without fear and birthing educators can focus on releasing stress that is unrelated to birthing itself.

In the meantime, we offer suggestions to help you get started so that as you thoroughly prepare, you can take steps that ensure that your birth experience is as healthy, safe, and positively memorable as possible.

• Educate yourself by reading as many positive approaches to birthing as you can. Your HypnoBirthing Practitioner can recommend reading that will support your positive outlook. I, of course, personally recommend the updated and edited version of <u>Childbirth Without Fear</u> by Dr. Grantly Dick-Read. Additionally, I suggest <u>The Birth Book</u> by Sears and Sears, for starters. Avoid books that focus on how to prepare yourself to face pain. Don't limit your education to stories that others feel compelled to impose upon you. Gently remind negative people that you are preparing for your birthing with HypnoBirthing and don't wish to engage in conversations that depict birth in a negative way.

• Interview potential medical caregivers to be sure that the one you select is supportive of your wishes for as little medical intervention as possible. If you are inquiring into a medical association, be sure that the entire medical team will honor your requests. Ask about their thinking on key issues like avoiding the use of Pitocin for artificial induction or labor augmentation, what their thinking is about allowing labor to run its course and what their C-section rate is. Most importantly, observe their reaction to your wanting to discuss your labor in advance. How comfortable are they with your thinking? Are they defensive, or are they pleased by your interest? You cannot leave these issues to chance, hoping that you and your doctor or midwife will see eye to eye when the time comes. Don't be afraid to assert yourself. You need to accept responsibility for your requests and for your decisions. My experience has been that clients who take the initiative in planning for birthing are very well received by their doctors and midwives, and particularly by attending nurses. Sometimes medical caregivers need just this gentle nudge to remind them of how they felt before they got caught up in the "busyness" of doing things routinely.

• Tour more than one birthing facility and talk with staff, just as you did when you selected your medical care provider. Find out how flexible they are and how willing they are to accommodate patient requests. The closest facility doesn't need to be your only option.

• Encourage your partner to attend classes with you, to read, and to take an active part in assisting with your practice. If you detect a reluctance, perhaps you should consider a secondary birthing companion for your labor and birthing. Both people will be welcome at your classes. It's not unusual for a partner to absolutely blossom when it comes down to actual labor, even if this wasn't the case beforehand--but you really can't bank on its happening. You may also arrange for your HypnoBirthing Practitioner to attend your birth. Most are happy to attend.

• If you've had a cesarean section previously, seriously consider having VBAC (vaginal birth after cesarean). According to the American

College of Obstetricians and Gynecologists VBAC Guidelines, October 1988, VBAC is safer in most cases than a scheduled repeat cesarean. Up to 80% of women are successful in birthing vaginally after a C-section. With HypnoBirthing, your relaxed attitude and prepared body could make a world of difference.

•    Ensure that you and your baby remain healthy by carefully selecting what you eat to be sure that you have a balanced diet. "Eating for two" doesn't mean that you eat ravenously; it refers to the care with which you select what you eat. Shed habits such as smoking, drinking, or using drugs during your pregnancy. They can be harmful to your developing baby. Your HypnoBirthing Practitioner can help you release these habits or can recommend a hypnotherapist to you.

•    Practice your slow breathing and the toning exercises that are described in a later chapter in this book and relax with your Rainbow Relaxation and Birthing Affirmations tapes daily. Your HypnoBirthing Practitioner will provide you with scripts that you and your birthing companion should practice with regularly. The success of your program depends on your following these prescribed activities.

*"Besides being a time for growing a baby, pregnancy is a time when you grow as a person, healing memories or fears about birth, working out a birthing philosophy. . . "*

*Sears & Sears*
*The Birth Book*

# The Curse of Eve

## The Origin of the Concept of Pain in Birthing

I include this sketchy account of the history of women and birthing, not to dwell on the negative past, but rather to offer it as an explanation of how birthing went awry and how we came to be where we are. Even more importantly, I feel it's vital that both women and men, medical caregivers, and lay persons, all understand that we no longer have to live with the sad legacy that these earlier times left to us; therefore, we no longer need to live with the fear of pain and suffering in birthing.

For centuries women have lived with faulty programming surrounding the nature of birthing, especially in Western society. Until a relatively short time ago, to even think of the word "natural" in connection with the birthing of a child was incongruous. For countless generations, women have expected, and have been expected, to go through agony during birthing; and when pain is expected, pain is experienced.

As regrettable as it may seem, the belief that pain is a natural accompaniment of birthing has actually been bestowed upon women. As we delve into the history of civilization (?), we learn that it was not always this way. Even today in some of the less sophisticated societies where people have not been influenced by Western Civilization, women with bodies that are physiologically identical to those of Western women, give birth with relatively no fanfare and with a minimum of discomfort. They have never been taught, nor learned to live with and accept, the horrors of "The Curse of Eve."

To understand the sequence of events that led to our present belief structure surrounding the "sorrow" with which women have supposedly been cursed, we have to look back to as early as 3,000 years before the birth of Christ and the spread of the Christian-Judeo doctrines--back to a time when women had their babies naturally and with a minimum of discomfort, unless there was complication. The lives of the people in these ancient times centered around Nature and motherhood. They honored Mother Nature, Mother Earth, and Mother Creator. Women were revered as the givers of life.

Because there was no awareness of the link between intercourse and the conception of a child, it was believed that women brought forth children at will. As creators, responsible for the survival of the human race, they were thought to be connected to deity. Statues of the goddesses of these early people were of full-breasted women with bodies clearly depicting the ballooning abdomen of women about to give birth. These primal people worshipped all of Nature and regarded birthing as the highest manifestation of Nature. When a woman was about to give birth, everyone gathered around her in the temple for the "celebration of life" to ask their deity to bless the child with health and strength. Birthing was a religious rite, and not at all the painful ordeal it was later to become.

Women were nurturers and healers. Whatever medicines were used were developed, brewed, and administered by women. They collaborated and exchanged their learning, often overseen by the "wise women" of the village. All healing was provided by the hands and the healing spirit of women. Men were the gatherers of food, herbs, and building materials. Their roles were different, yet equal.

A joyous attitude toward birthing prevailed for many centuries, and study shows that the Grecian School of medicine, led by Hippocrates and Aristotle, gave no indication in their writings that there was pain associated with childbirth, except in the event of a complication. Even then, women were brought into a relaxed state with herbs and brews so that the complication could be treated. While the Greeks recognized a male god as supreme, they gave equal stature to both men and women in their lesser gods; and women enjoyed a position of respect at the center of their religion.

Both Hippocrates and Aristotle believed that the needs and the feelings of women in childbirth were to be accommodated. They advocated having support persons attend a laboring woman. Hippocrates was the first to organize and give formal instruction to women who engaged in midwifery.

Hippocrates and Aristotle repeatedly wrote that Nature is the best physician and that it (Nature) should be allowed to function without the intrusion of ". . . meddlesome interference." Aristotle wrote of the mind-body connection in his teachings and emphasized the importance of deep relaxation during childbirth. Neither wrote of pain in his notes on normal birthing.

Just 79 years before the birth of Christ, another from the Grecian School, Soranus, began to put the writings of Aristotle and Hippocrates into book form. Soranus' contribution earned him the reputation of having been the greatest obstetrical man of the times. He stressed the importance of listening to the needs and feelings of women giving birth and advocated using the powers of the mind to achieve relaxation to bring about easy birthing. Like Aristotle and Hippocrates, Soranus included no mention of pain, except when he wrote of abnormal or complicated birth. On these occasions, he, too, recommended the use of herbs and brews to relieve discomfort. Women were treated kindly, gently, and joyfully during the natural occasion of giving birth.

Some of this approach to childbirth lasted for hundreds of years in Greece. As recent as the 1930s, women in small rural areas of Greece gathered around a "birthing tree"--a tree with low branches to which a laboring mother could cling as she expelled her baby during the second stage of labor. Joy was the prevailing emotion, not fear or sorrow.

This philosophy did not prevail throughout the rest of Europe, however. As tribes began to conquer and expand their holdings, war became glorified, and warriors were held up as leaders. With the spread of Christianity, a new belief began to take hold in Europe, and it brought with it "The Curse of Eve." The belief in a single, male god left no room for the goddess concept. The stone temples and altars of the people who worshipped Nature were destroyed, and Christian cathedrals sprang up in their place. The statues of their gods, those womanly icons, were smashed and buried. To ascribe any importance to the laws or functions of Nature became a serious offense, and all writings dealing with natural cures were seized and buried. Regrettably, Soranus' books on natural birthing met the same sad fate.

In an effort to make the new religion more palatable, many of the Nature worshipers' traditions, symbols, and festivals were retained. Their winter solstice festival, at the darkest time of the year, remained, along with the symbols of Nature--the yule logs, trees, mistletoe, and holly used in their celebrations. These symbols are still prevalent today at the Christmas season, as are their symbols of fertility--the rabbit, the egg, and the chick, which were revered at the time of their "Easterly Celebration" when the breezes from the East came to warm the earth in preparation for sowing.

The role of women in religion and society most assuredly did not remain. Literally, few stones were left unturned as they set out to crush the goddess concept and redefine the role of women. In the second century St. Clement of Alexandria wrote: "Every woman should be filled with shame by the thought that she is a woman." Poor and uneducated women became afraid simply to be women. They were forbidden to practice their healing arts, forced to meet in secrecy, and able to work only by dark of night. Hence, witchcraft, which previously had been an honorable, healing gift, was denounced as a tool of the devil and banned. All matters of medicine and healing were placed firmly into the hands of priests and monks, who claimed their power as a directive from God. The clergy exercised complete authority over decisions as to who would be treated and who wouldn't.

Blamed for the fall from grace and for every illness and misfortune that occurred as a result, hundreds of thousands of peasant women were declared witches and were systematically executed by prolonged torture, mutilation, and burning at the stake--their alleged crime being their ability to both cause illnesses and, conversely, to effect cures. Since Church doctrine ordained that only God had the power to cure, their successes in healing proved that they were, indeed, in collaboration with the devil. This travesty continued for more than five centuries, with women and girl children of entire villages being put to death. Bounties were paid to people who would expose the healer witches and to those who would drag them to the center of the village to be executed. Many were willing to accuse and deliver.

The largest number of executions took place in Germany, with as many as four hundred deaths by execution being performed in a single day. Those who escaped execution were branded outcasts, were looked upon as inferiors, and were relegated to lives of subserviency. It is written that their ignorance created their subserviency, and their subserviency created their ignorance. Others, in order to survive, denied their healing skills and submitted to the authority of the Church. The translations of the Hebrew account of creation made it very clear that women were to be subjugated in their relationships with their husbands and in society in general.

Men in medicine, government, and in the Church waged an all-out effort to eradicate the image of women and birthing being the focus of religious celebration. The effort was successful. By a series of decrees that extended over centuries, what had been a celebration of life eroded into an excruciatingly painful, lonely, and much-to-be-feared ordeal. Law demanded that women be segregated during pregnancy and isolated during birthing. With authority over all medical practice and healing firmly ensconced in the hands of the priests and monks, doctors had to obtain permission to administer to "the deserving ill." Since children were the result of "carnal sin," women in labor were not considered among the deserving ill. People in the medical field were forbidden to attend a woman in labor. This ensured that even in the event of a complicated birth, no drugs or herbs could be administered to a laboring woman. Midwifery was abolished, leaving the laboring mother isolated and without support.

Citing the need for women to pay retribution for original sin, there was a deaf ear turned to pleas for mercy. Women who experienced labors that were complicated suffered untold horrors. New laws demanded that if there were complication, a live baby was to be taken. In such an event, field hands and goat gelders, the only people allowed to attend a woman in labor, "took" the baby by cutting through the wall of the uterus, with no regard for the life or agony of the mother. If a live baby could not be taken, it was mandated that the baby be baptized in the womb by the same method. Women who died were considered "saved" for having brought a new soul into the world. Women paid the price of original sin, and it was, indeed, a high one.

It was here that a belief structure that has endured for centuries took hold--women must endure excruciating pain in bringing children into the world.

When we look back upon these events, we understand that it was fear of complication and resulting death, not fear of birthing, that caused women to look upon labor with horror. Extreme fear created extreme tension; and the tension, in turn, resulted in a taut cervix, unable to perform its natural function. Those who lived through the ordeal, as well as those who witnessed it, attested to the agony that was experienced in birthing.

It's impossible to even think that a woman could approach the birthing experience with anything but the most terrifying fear, knowing that in the event of a complication, at best, she would experience outrageous suffering; and at worst, she may never live through the ordeal. It was very clear that birthing was no longer considered a celebration of life. In the eyes of Church and community leaders and, indeed, in the eyes and minds of women themselves, a painful birthing was the sentence that women were to endure throughout eternity. The Fear-Tension-Pain Syndrome was deeply established, and it created its own continuum.

Medicine advanced with the rebirth of science after the dark and middle ages, but the status of women and birthing did not. Biblical translations, written at a time when it was believed that pain was a natural accompaniment of birthing, kept the concept of "The Curse of Eve" alive. Through his study into the Bible and from his association with scholars of the Bible, Dick-Read learned that the Hebrew word <u>etzev</u> is translated to mean "labor, toil, and work" throughout most bibles; but when the same translators referred to childbirth, the word was given to mean "pain, sorrow, anguish, or pangs." Still other scholars point out that the prophets made no such references in their writings on childbirth.

It was many centuries before there was any breakthrough in attitude surrounding women, healing, and birthing. From the 13th to the 16th centuries, women, branded as witches, continued to be executed for their role as healers.

Finally, in the early 16th Century, the lost writings of Soranus were discovered. The medical world took interest, and those in medicine who were driven by conscience defied the existing laws. The first book on obstetrics was written, based on the theories and teachings of the most profound medical philosophers and practitioners the world had yet known.

Only in the latter part of the 16th Century were herdsmen and shepherds prohibited by law from attending women in labor; but, still, physicians were not able to attend in the birthing process.

At this time, midwifery came back into practice, but it was looked upon as a dishonorable occupation, ". . .best suited to women to take care of the nasty business of giving birth." In Germany, where the largest number of executions of women occurred, Martin Luther wrote, ". . . If women become tired or even die, it does not matter. Let them die in childbirth. That's what they are there for." He conceived a title for midwives that expressed the prevailing beliefs of the time and, in itself, suggested pain. "Weh mutters," literally translated from the German, "weh" (pain) and "mutter" (mother), "Mothers of woe," was the name he attached to the women who attended birthing mothers.

Even with the advent of chloroform, there was no relief for the birthing mother. Its use was forbidden during childbirth, though it was permitted for all other medical procedures. This attitude toward women and birthing was not limited to Europe. A New England minister, when it was suggested that relief be given to women in labor, responded that to do so would rob God of the pleasure of their, ". . .deep, earnest cries for help."

It wasn't until well into the middle of the 18th Century that doctors were allowed to attend women. Even then, doctors who practiced obstetrics were usually inept and/or alcoholics. Maternity hospitals were appallingly dirty. Infections from something as simple as unwashed hands ran rampant. Some women who gave birth at home died of complication, but many more who went to hospitals for safety and good treatment died from infection called "childbed fever." Though the deaths were a result of lack of sanitation rather than a complicated birth, fear of death became even more strongly associated with giving birth.

Much of the credit for improved conditions belongs to Florence Nightingale, an influential woman of wealth. Nightingale insisted that maternity wards adopt the same standards of sanitation and cleanliness as other wards in hospitals; and, using her money as clout, she saw to it that the inept, alcoholic doctors disappeared from the birthing scene. Because of her influence, standards of training and practice were also raised. With the changes that Nightingale brought about, the number of mothers succumbing to childbed fever declined to an almost nonexistent level.

Very little was done to effect change in birthing practice for many years. Widespread knowledge of anesthetics, hygiene, antibiotics, and pain relievers was not evident until the 1900s. Before that, the agony of a woman in labor was incredible. Eventually, pressure from influential people brought about a softer attitude, and the use of anesthesia was allowed during birthing. Once the door was opened to the use of anesthesia, the pendulum swung very quickly to the opposite end. Early administration of drugs and anesthesia became the standard for all deliveries and labors. Since it was believed that painful delivery was inevitable, women were given heavy doses of pain killers during the first stage of labor and were administered general anesthesia as soon as there was any indication of crowning. Drugged births, where babies were pulled from the birth canal with instruments, became the rule. Relief for the woman and expediency for the medical staff ruled the day and, to some extent, still does.

Even though Grantly Dick-Read forwarded his theory as early as 1920 and throughout the 30s and 40s and into the 50s, the effects of drugs on both the mother and the child during labor didn't become a matter of concern until the late 60s. Out of that concern came efforts to teach women how to cope with the pain of labor. Because large numbers of women were successfully giving birth without having been administered drugs, the term "Natural Childbirth" was used to describe the procedure, but huffing and puffing a child into the world hardly holds up a mirror to nature.

Natural childbirth is still relatively young, but the belief that labor is a painful experience has had centuries to become imbedded in the minds of women and men alike, including medical caregivers.

There is still much work to be done, for an incredible number of doctors, midwives, childbirth educators, health care providers, and obstetric nurses reinforce the pain concept through their choice of words and advice during childbirth education classes and in labor rooms. Women themselves still believe that there must of necessity be pain in childbirth and that the best they can do is learn how to survive it, rather than learn how to alleviate it. Artificial inducement and augmentation of labor is creating a slippery slope whereby additional drugs may be necessary to quell the pain brought on by the first drug. Collaborative, natural techniques to initiate or augment labor are being ignored. It doesn't have to be that way.

Through self-hypnosis, relaxation, and natural techniques taught in HypnoBirthing classes, we can move forward (or backward, as the case may be) and replace fear and anxiety with confidence, serenity, happiness, and celebration. In learning this most natural birthing method, you will find that you have so many options. Learning to allow your mind, your body, and your baby to work together in natural harmony can provide for you the safe and satisfying birthing that you seek.

*". . .knowing your body, reading its signals, and trusting your responses. Therein lie the keys to a positive birth experience."*

*William & Martha Sears*
*The Birth Book*

# What's Wrong with Labor?

Occasionally one of the women in a HypnoBirthing class will ask, "Why don't we human beings have our babies the way cats and dogs and horses and other animals do?" My reply is always the same: "Yes, why don't we?"

When we examine a premise held by medical professionals, we learn that pain is considered "the watchdog of medicine." Pain, they tell us, sends a signal that something is wrong.

Each day we perform countless numbers of tasks using muscles in every way imaginable. We lift our legs and move our hips to climb stairs; we raise our arms, move our fingers, blink our eyes. We ingest food, digest it, and expel it--all without difficulty. We perform all of these moves and more; yet, we feel no discomfort. It is only when something is wrong--when we perform these tasks with a wrong twist or turn, or when something is pathologically wrong, that pain is experienced. All of this begs the question, WHAT'S WRONG WITH LABOR?

Most women who have given birth will emphatically state that what's wrong with labor is pain. Labor hurts. Too many couples come away from their birthing experience with birth stories that are tinged with apology and disappointment as they speak of long periods of terrible pain, drugs, and feelings of helplessness. That being the case, we must again ask the question, "Why is pain experienced in labor?" WHAT'S WRONG WITH LABOR? How can it be that women, with bodies so perfectly created to conceive, nurture, and birth a baby, experience pain during labor.

Prominent doctors--heads of obstetrical departments at medical schools--have written articles on why labor hurts and state that what creates discomfort in labor is that there are two sets of muscles that work in resistance to each other. While that may be what often happens in labor, we are still left with the question, "Why do these particular two sets of muscles work in opposition?" WHAT'S WRONG WITH LABOR?

Most Western women are in awe of women from less urbanized areas and underdeveloped countries of the world because of the ease with which they bring children into the world, without pain or anesthesia. What do they know about labor that we in our more sophisticated, highly technological part of the world have not yet learned? Specifically, we need to ask, WHAT'S WRONG WITH OUR LABORS?

It was in a humble, poverty-ridden setting in London in 1913 that

Grantly Dick-Read first became sensitive to the possible answer to what is wrong with labor. As a young intern in London's White Chapel District in the heart of the East End slums, he was called to attend a woman in labor. After traveling on his bicycle through mud and rain, he arrived about three in the morning at a low hovel underneath some railroad arches. He found his way to a small apartment, where he discovered his patient in a dim room, soaked from the rain that was pouring in on her. She was covered with only sacks and an old black skirt. He asked permission to put the mask over her face and administer chloroform. Her emphatic refusal was a first for Dick-Read. He returned his things to his bag, stood back, and watched. Her baby was born with no fuss and with no noise from the patient. As he prepared to leave, Dick-Read asked why she had refused the relief from pain. She gave him an answer that he was never to forget--"It didn't hurt. It wasn't meant to, was it, Doctor?"--an honest answer, given in a deep cockney accent, that has had a profound effect on birthing for many decades.

The significance of relaxed birthing, free of the intrusive fear and the resulting constrictors, became increasingly obvious to Dick-Rick in the months that followed, as he sat with more affluent, laboring women in the London Hospital--women who experienced both agony and terror throughout labor and birthing. He mentally compared these patients with the tranquil, calm, and comfortable woman in the hovel and asked,"Why?"

Similar experiences presented themselves to Dick-Read when he was in the service during World War I. On a battlefield in a foreign land, a woman, very much in labor, approached a trench, asking for a doctor. She was helped down into the trench where Dick-Read was on duty, and she proceeded to give birth, apparently with no discomfort and completely oblivious to the war going on around her. When she was finished, she wrapped her baby and went on her way.

On another occasion he encountered a laboring woman, propped against an embankment, giving birth. The baby arrived easily. He watched as she waited, holding the baby in her arms. He could see that the umbilicus began to thin, like a string. The woman then proceeded to either tear or cut the cord with her fingernails. Having completed her task, she started her journey back to her village, her newborn in her arms.

It was these events that prompted Dick-Read to rethink his beliefs and what he had been taught about birthing. With these experiences behind him, he embarked into years of study. From this study came his theory that in the absence of fear during labor, the pain-causing constrictors are not prevalent, and the uterus is able to naturally efface, open, swell rhythmically, and expel the baby with ease.

As early as in the 1920s Dick-Read forwarded the answer to the question, WHAT'S WRONG WITH LABOR? when he presented his theory on the Fear-Tension-Pain Syndrome. No one was listening. His method later gained some attention with the publication of his book, Natural Childbirth, in 1933. Unfortunately, his colleagues, accustomed to "conducting deliveries" with drugs and forceps, still were not listening. The theory that there was something within our bodies that, in the absence of tension, released a natural anesthesia seemed rather radical at the time.

In the 1950s the second printing of his book, Revelations on Childbirth was published in the States under the title Childbirth Without Fear. For those of us who didn't buy into the generally accepted "something's-naturally-wrong-with-labor concept," he became our hero.

Even today, when women who used the Dick-Read method meet, there is an instant comradery. There is a feeling of having been among an "elite" few. We learned from his writings that what's wrong with labor has nothing to do with our physiology; and, when we were given proper preparation, our labors could unfold as they were intended. We followed his philosophy, practiced his breathing techniques, totally relaxed, let our bodies work naturally, and had pain-free birthings.

Simply put, we learned that what's wrong with labor takes place long before a woman goes into labor. It starts with FEAR--all of the fear that is so thoroughly ingrained in the minds of women as they approach their time of birthing. Even though the circumstances of the early historical events surrounding birthing no longer exist, a strong belief in pain is still held by most healthcare providers, birthing educators, and women themselves. Fear has been perpetuated, and it has become a self-fulfilling continuum--pain is expected, fear is prevalent, the body is tense, and pain is experienced.

Some motivational speakers refer to the word "fear" as an acronym: F-False, E-Evidence, A-Assuming, R-Reality; and nothing could be closer to the truth when it comes to labor.

It's easy to understand how this fear could exist. From the time little girls are old enough to understand and be included in adult conversation about birthing, they clearly learn that there is much to be feared in having a baby. Even the most positive-thinking mother-to-be, almost from the very start of her pregnancy, finds herself inundated with comments and advice about all of the things to watch out for and be careful of. These are well-intended dictums, but they contain the hidden message, "Be scared! Be afraid." Most pronouncements are of a warning nature, designed to put her on guard--as though they are preparing her for all of the hardships of pregnancy and labor that she will have to endure. Even in some medical offices, a woman who expresses optimism and confidence that she can have a gentle birth is immediately told the "error" of her thinking.

In addition to having the power to cut through the joy and anticipation that the mother is feeling, these kinds of conversations also have the ability to plant seeds of fear that can make the difference between a calm, serene birthing and a tense, painful ordeal.

As you work through this program, you will gain a better understanding of this philosophy. You will find yourself growing in confidence as you watch films of beautifully peaceful HypnoBirthings. Your willingness to practice and prepare your mind and body to work in complete harmony will ultimately lead to that safe, beautiful birth experience that you have come to believe in and expect. You will have eliminated the fear that is at the root of WHAT'S WRONG WITH LABOR.

*"You see things as they are, and you ask, 'Why?' But I see things as they could be; and I ask, 'Why not?'"*

*(Paraphrase) George Bernard Shaw*
*Back to Methuselah*

---

# *Your Marvelous Birthing Device--The Uterus*

---

At first glance, it may appear that any discussion of how the uterus functions is out of place in this segment of your birthing course. It is important, however, to devote time and space to this topic at this point because of its relationship to fear and pain. We must understand the way in which the uterus functions naturally in order to understand how fear can throw a monkey wrench into the workings of this smooth birthing muscle.

With this knowledge in hand, the concept of easier, more comfortable childbirth becomes immediately obvious and, therefore, attainable. This very brief and simple explanation that follows is, indeed, the crux of the entire program.

You will want to be sure that you fully understand this concept, as it is exactly this process of your body that you will work with during labor.

## The Uterine Layers

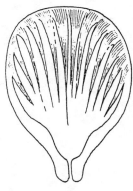

The outer longitudinal
muscle fibers

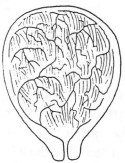

The middle muscle layers,
interwoven with blood vessels

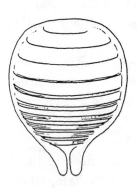

The inner circular muscle
layers found mostly at the
lower part of the uterus

There are three layers of muscle in the uterus. The two layers with which we will be concerned are the outer layer, with muscles that are vertical, and the inner layer, with muscles that are horizontally circular.

The illustrations on the previous page show the three sets of muscle layers within the uterus and the concentration of the working muscles in the two layers that are actually involved in birthing.

The circular muscles of the inner layer are found in the lower portion of the uterus. As the illustrations show, the circular muscles are thickest just above the opening, or neck, of the uterus. In order for the outlet of the uterus to open and permit the baby to easily move down, through, and out of the uterus into the birth canal, these thicker muscles have to be drawn up and back.

The stronger muscles at the top of the outer layer of the uterus are vertical fibers. They go up the back and over the top of the uterus, drawing up the relaxed circular muscles. In an almost wavelike motion, these long muscle bands shorten and flex to push the baby down, through, and ultimately out of the uterus.

When the laboring mother is in a comfortable state of relaxation, the two sets of muscles work in harmony, as they were intended to. The surge of the vertical muscles draws up, flexes, and expels; and the circular muscles open and draw back to allow this to happen. Birthing then goes smoothly and easily.

The techniques you will learn in the HypnoBirthing Program and the relaxation practice you will do on a daily basis at home will teach you how to work with these birthing muscles for easier labor.

# How Fear Affects Labor

## CATECHOLAMINE--THE ENEMY OF THE LABOR ROOM

Fear--one of the strongest emotions that we know--is, indeed, a villain in the labor room. When we experience stress, messages are sent to all of the receptors in the body, creating exaggerated and distorted reactions. These amplified messages then create physiological and chemical changes within the body. When the body is put on the defensive, the stress hormones--catecholamines--are triggered so that we immediately experience a "fight or flight" response. These hormones play a major role in the body's physiological response.

When circumstances are such that neither "fight" nor "flight" are appropriate options, as in the case of a laboring mother, catecholamines act as constrictors, causing the muscles within the uterus and elsewhere to tense. It is believed that catecholamine is released in large concentration prior to and during labor when a woman approaches birthing with unresolved fear.

Simply put, fear affects sensations that are felt throughout the body and puts the body into a state of alert. To protect itself when it is in a state of defense, the body directs all possible effort to those areas that can assist in the "fight" or the "flight." Since the uterus plays no part in the body's defense, the focus is to send blood to other organs and muscles by constricting the arteries going to the uterus. If this occurs over a short period of time, there is little harmful effect; however, limited oxygen in the uterus for a prolonged period of time can be detrimental to the baby. The lack of blood flow to the uterus also results in a constricting of the muscles so that instead of relaxing and opening, the circular fibers at the neck of the uterus tighten. When this happens, the vertical muscles continue to try to draw the circular muscles up and back; but the cervix is resistent.

In addition to creating considerable pain for the laboring mother when these two sets of muscles work in opposition, the situation can also have an adverse effect on the baby. As the vertical muscles push to expel, the taut neck of the cervix refuses to budge. The baby's head is then forced against an unrelenting, constricted muscle. When the laboring mother is consciously (or subconsciously) fearful, she is inwardly tense, labor is lengthened, and pain is created.

You and your birthing companion will be taught how to identify emotional stress before and during labor, how to release it, and how to bring yourself into a deepened relaxation. When you are confident and free of fear, you can bring yourself into a calm, relaxed state from the very onset of labor. Your birthing companion will lend support to this relaxation. Verbal and physical cues that you and your partner have practiced will initially bring you into a state of calm so that the constricting hormones are overridden by your body's natural relaxants, endorphins.

The extended relaxation tape that you will practice with daily allows the uterus to remain in a relaxed state most of the time, leaving room for the baby to turn later in anticipation of birth. Only a very few HypnoBirthing mothers experience breech presentation of their babies. (See "When Baby is Breech" on Page 102.)

## ENDORPHINS--THE BODY'S NATURAL PAIN KILLERS

Dick-Read was more than a half century ahead of his time. He didn't put a name to it, but he knew from observation that when laboring mothers were free of fear, their bodies relaxed; the muscles of their cervix relaxed; and something wonderful happened that permitted an easier birth.

Scientists have long searched for alternatives to pain-killing drugs; but it wasn't until sometime in the 70s that it was discovered that the source of natural analgesic lies within the body itself. Studying the way in which opiates work upon the body, American researchers discovered that opiate molecules, locking onto special receptor sites of neurons in the central nervous system, slowed down the firing rate of the neurons. They found that if they decreased the firing rate of the neurons, it resulted in a decrease in the sensation of pain. Many of these neurons are located in the spinal cord, where pain is eventually processed into an actual bodily sensation.

With this information behind them, it was not long before scientists isolated **Endorphins**--neuropeptides in the brain and pituitary gland which have an effect that is 200 times that of morphine. Because they suppress synaptic activity that leads to pain sensation, endorphins produce a tranquil, amnesiac condition. At that same time, smaller, breakdown products of endorphins, called enkephalins, which literally means "in the head," were discovered.

What to Dick-Read was observation and theory in the 20s became founded in scientific research and discovery in the 70s. In the 1920s when no one knew of the existence of the body's own natural analgesics, it was inconceivable to think of alleviating pain through relaxation. Few of Dick-Read's colleagues would even consider the premise that the uterine muscles used in childbirth could work harmoniously and that labor could be painless. The concept of painful labor was very thoroughly embedded. Dick-Read was disappointed, but not defeated. He continued to study and to do further writing on his Fear-Tension-Pain Syndrome.

Regrettably, he did not live long enough to see his theory buttressed as a result of the discovery of endorphins. Still more regrettable is that, even with this discovery in hand, too few medical caregivers are considering the effect that endorphins have on birthing. Its application is finding its way into labor rooms and childbirth education classrooms at only a snail's pace.

Through relaxation, self-hypnosis, and guided imagery taught in HypnoBirthing classes, you will be able to create a path to the center of the subconscious and tap these natural tranquilizers--endorphins--thus alleviating the pain-causing hormone, catecholamine, before it starts.

*"Contractions don't have to hurt. They are energy rushes that enable you to open up your thing so the baby can come out. If you have the attitude that they hurt, then you'll tense up and not be able to relax, and it will take the baby longer to come through and you won't have any fun either."*

*Barbara*
*Spiritual Midwifery*

# Releasing Fear

Preparing women for birthing by educating them in the physiology of labor clearly teaches that birthing muscles are designed to give birth smoothly.

For many women in the 50s that appeal to their intellect was enough to cause them to break with the traditional attitudes of our culture and to bring their children into the world using the techniques of Natural Childbirth. They were free of all fear of labor and, consequently, free of the discomfort of labor.

For many others, however, even though they embraced the premise, did the exercises, learned the breathing techniques, and approached labor without fear, their labors were only slightly easier than those of their sisters who had traditional births. They addressed their fear of labor, but they neglected to consider the impact of other emotions on pregnancy and labor.

Like most other women, you will find that your pregnancy brings with it a whole new set of feelings, anxieties, doubts, questions, decisions, and tasks that you never had to consider before. Some of these will center around your labor and birthing, but many more will cause you to look at the many changes that bringing a baby into your life will present. You will want to be ready in this regard also--free of any fears or reservations.

It's important that you identify feelings, experiences, or recollections that may be painful or hurtful. Take a look at those emotions that may foster a feeling of uneasiness, meet them head on, and release any conflict you may be harboring (consciously or subconciously) because of them. Once you have been able to work through and resolve lingering emotions that could stand in the way of an easier birthing, you will have a better sense of your own ability to approach the birth of your baby with trust and confidence.

You will want to thoroughly search your inner feelings to discover the areas that you feel very confident about and those that you need to work through so that you can resolve any fears or misgivings that you are holding. Brushing aside the matters of concern to you may help you to get through your pregnancy; but they can easily surface as fears when you are in labor, and they can affect the course of your labor. You may want to ask your partner or your birthing companion or a good friend to sit down with you so that you can explore and discuss some of the thoughts that could be troubling you.

Your HypnoBirthing Practitioner will provide you with an inventory that will assist you in identifying those areas of your life that you need to work through and will work with you in fear release sessions in class. If after you do the sessions in class and talk with your partner and friends, you still feel you need some assistance in releasing lingering fears, ask your practitioner for a private session. If you are not able to work with a trained practitioner, you may find it helpful to seek the counsel of a hypnotherapist to do release work with you. A fear release hypnotherapy session is truly one of the most effective ways of eliminating toxic emotions.

Listed below are just a few of the areas of concern to pregnant women that surfaced in the early 90s as a result of the Dr. Lewis Mehl study on turning breech babies with hypnosis and other research. Your own inventory may reveal other issues that you need to resolve.

- **Your own birth**--What are the stories that you have heard about your own birth? Are they positive and encouraging, or negative and frightening? Do you feel that you will duplicate your mother's labor?

- **Other birth stories**--Have you been surrounded with stories of joyful birthing, or have family members impressed upon you "family patterns" of long labors, back labor, severe pain, and medical intervention?

- **Previous labors**--Has your own experience with labor been easy and satisfying, or are you carrying recollections of an arduous ordeal?

- **Parenting**--Did you learn positive attitudes toward parenting that you feel comfortable with? If not, do you feel less than adequate about your ability to be a good parent? Do you feel overwhelmed?

- **Support**--Do you feel secure with the support that your partner and/or family will provide? Is there someone who will share the responsibilities of taking care of the baby?

- **Marriage/relationship**--Is your marriage/relationship a secure, loving, and mutually nurturing relationship? Are you confident that your relationship is strong and that it will weather the additional concerns of raising a child? Are there some agreements you need to work out? Have you "talked?"

- **Career**--Will you be able to continue to pursue your own goals with reorganizing and planning? Will your plans need to be put on hold?

- **Housing**--Is there room in your home, as well as in your heart, for your new baby? Can accommodations be easily made?

- **Medical care**--Do you feel comfortable with your present medical care provider? Do you feel that he or she is supportive of your plans for your birthing?

- **Finances**--Do you see finances being "stretched" as a result of adding another person into your life?

- **Prior relationships**--Are you carrying around unhappy memories of an earlier relationship or an experience that has left hurtful thoughts?

Your HypnoBirthing Practitioner will gladly help you clear any concerns that you may have. It's important that you approach your birthing as free of "emotional baggage" as you can be.

*"Mothers-to-be have long believed that they influence their babies by what they do and how they do it."*

*T. Berry Brazelton. M.D.*

# *Prenatal Bonding*

## *"A Womb with a View"*

A fairly new study, fetology, is drawing a considerable amount of attention. This branch of medicine focuses on the effects of environment upon the developing fetus. Attempts are being made to determine the degree to which a baby in the uterus is affected by the environment in which he is living and the manner in which his parents interact with him. Gaining more acceptance is the belief that while your baby is growing and developing physically, it is also developing emotionally and psychically. Influences, both good and bad, are imprinting.

One of the pioneers in this field, a Canadian doctor named Thomas Verney, began his research in the mid-to-late 70s. Much has been written since that bears out the suspicion that it is important to be aware of the kind of environment and experiences you are providing to your unborn child. On the negative side, it was noted that the pulse rate of the fetus rises abruptly when the child is exposed to screaming, yelling, loud or disturbing noises, and emotional upsets. Additionally, these emotional tugs of war can cause an upset mother to smoke or drink or in other ways create an atmosphere that is not conducive to relaxation and the emotional or physical well being of the baby.

As a result of Verney's studies and those of his contemporaries who picked up on his work, it was found that babies in the womb can react to stimuli outside of the uterus. Intentionally initiating certain kinds of interaction can result in positive prenatal, perinatal, and postnatal bonding.

Findings suggest that babies within the womb react to:

vibrations • stroking • tapping • rubbing • squeezing
conversation • voices • music • light • heat • cold
pressing to simulate the birth experience • teasing
loud noises • TV sounds • humor

It was found that babies who were exposed to soft music and singing during gestation were calmer and they adjusted more easily. As a result, they were better sleepers.

From a study by Dr. Michael Lazarev, a leading Russian pediatrician, it was noted that parents who interact with their unborn babies through music definitely will find a response from the fetus. He stresses the importance of helping the baby to become familiar with musical sounds both before it is born and while it is an infant. Lazarev concluded that if you listen to your baby, it will let you know what activities and sounds it prefers.

One Russian woman in the Lazarev study reported that when she was 37 weeks pregnant, she attended a rock concert but had to leave the concert because the baby was kicking so furiously, she felt she was going to be sick. Another reported that if she listened to Rachmaninoff and visualized swimming, the baby began to move in a soft swirling manner.

A couple who responded to the study told of engaging in an argument. Their baby began to react in a way that let them know that it wasn't comfortable with their tone. Still another woman reported that her baby would not allow her to type. As soon as she began to work at her typewriter, the baby began to become extremely active in an upsetting way. A woman who used to read fairy tales to her baby could sense by the kind of movement within the uterus that her baby was enjoying the stories.

Dr. Gerhand Rottman, of the University of Salzburg, forwarded his beliefs that positive interaction is beneficial to baby and parents. The mothers involved in interacting with their babies had a better attitude toward their own increasing size and displayed a more acceptant, and even proud, air about the shapes their bodies were taking on. Fathers displayed the same kind of respect and awe for the changes that were taking place in the mother. There was a respect for the life being carried in the womb. Overall, their pregnancies seemed to be easier, as were their birthings. They approached birthing with a relaxed confidence. Later, both parents seemed to adopt a softer, more balanced attitude toward care giving. Parents displayed greater feelings of enjoyment, love, and respect.

The benefits to babies were also profound. There were fewer premature births and fewer low-birth-weight babies. Reports showed a noticeable increase in the socialization of the babies who experienced prenatal bonding. Overall health and weight gain was very positive.

*"Let the sound awaken every cell of its being, echoing the harmony of nature."*
*Michael Lazarev, M.D., <u>Sonatal</u>*

# Recommendations for Prenatal Bonding

A. Learn relaxation techniques and practice them daily--baby needs peace too.

B. "Play" with baby physically--shake, shake, shake; rub, rub, rub; pat, pat, pat; squeeze, squeeze, squeeze; press, press, press (gently).

C. Use guided imagery and visualization. (See A Father's Script.)

D. Carry on conversations with baby--say affirmations, read stories with animation and imitation of animal sounds, play children's tapes.

E. Massage your abdomen with luke-warm water.

F. Play soothing music--ocean, birds, wind, soft piano, guitar, madrigals, flute, harp, etc.

G. Have family and friends greet and interact with baby.

H. Put yourself in the baby's frame of reference--how wholesome are the surrounding noises, voices, attitudes, emotions, foods, temperatures, air, odors?

*"If a mother fights with others while she is pregnant, the baby will come out fighting in childbirth, causing much pain. The baby will grow up fighting and arguing.*

*"Rogu from Mamatoto*

# *Prenatal Bonding Exercise*

What your baby perceives--what it accepts and embraces while in the uterus--becomes part of its essence and its identity and forms the creation of a conscious ego that accepts, caresses, and acknowledges its own true self.

Imagine that you are the baby that is developing within your mother's womb, listening to conversations, experiencing your surroundings, absorbing emotions and moods of those around you. Reflect for a few minutes on how you feel as that child who is about to be born.

- How welcome do you feel?
- How loved do you feel?
- What kinds of messages are you receiving from things that are said?
- What are your feelings about the interaction between your parents?
- What kind of pace do your parents keep? Will there be time purposely created for you?
- What kind of atmosphere will you come into?
- How confident are you that you will be raised with love and patience?
- How calm a world is being prepared for you?
- How loving are the people you will be living with?
- What tone of voice will be used by the people around you?
- Do the people you are going to live with talk in gentle, loving ways?
- Is each motion that you make received with joy?
- What kinds of sounds/music/noises do you live with?
- Is the nourishment that you are receiving conducive to your healthy growth?

- How wholesome is the air that you are breathing?  Will it foster good health for you?
- Is your environment and your body smoke free, alcohol free, and drug free?
- How certain are you that you will be helped and guided toward becoming a loved and loving human being?
- What kind of assurance do you have that your parents will give you understanding as you learn to adjust to your strange, new world?
- Are you confident that you will learn by guidance, not punishment?

Reflecting on your responses to these questions, are there some changes that you feel you can make in your baby's environment?  Are there some resolutions that you, as parents, need to think about and adopt?

*"Leave it to a baby to turn your world upside down, take your breath away, and make you fall in love again.  With his toothless grin, your baby sets your heart on fire."*

*Jan Blaustone*
*The Joy of Parenthood*

# A Father's Script

The birthing companion today is an active participant throughout the birthing experience. Rather than an onlooker who vacillates between feeling helpless and unknowledgeable, in HypnoBirthing the birth companion is actually the trained facilitator and primary support person for the birthing mother. The perinatal bonding that takes place among the mother, the baby, and the birthing companion during this wonderful interlude, combined with the mother's conditioned relaxation, is the whole key to achieving a more natural, easier, and sometimes even painless, birthing.

I adapted the following script from one that was originally composed by Henry Leo Bolduc in his book, Self-Hypnosis--Creating your Own Destiny. When I first read Henry's script, I was overwhelmed by the beauty of his words. I was particularly attracted to it because, in effect, it is an outpouring of the awe with which a father views this wonderful miracle. Henry expresses a sensitivity to perinatal bonding when he points out that the attitude and philosophy of the mother and the birthing companion are as much a gentle suggestion for the child during birthing as it is reassurance for the mother. With gratitude to Henry for giving me permission to incorporate a few HypnoBirthing images into his script, I include the following adaptation in the HypnoBirthing Program:

*New life is forming, growing, and moving within you. You are part of the promise and the destiny of life itself. A very important event is taking place in your life . . . a wonderfully normal, natural, biological, and spiritual event. You're going to have a baby. What is happening now is the process of birthing and freeing the kicking, moving little being who's been a part of your body for so long.*

*Soon it will be time for the baby to become its own separate person. One cycle is ending; and, immediately, another is beginning. What has been called "labor" is that in-between experience . . . the fulcrum . . . that small, short period of time and space between the baby's two worlds.*

*Change from one stage to another brings pressure, and then release. You will soon experience this as the change is completed and fulfilled. You can feel this and embrace it and welcome it as refreshing and totally natural.*

*With mind, you build a healthy attitude and happy expectation. Happy childbirth has much to do with a healthy, joyous, loving anticipation. It is something remarkably beautiful. Being a channel of new life is said to be a spiritual experience. With this understanding, total relaxation, and serene breathing, all discomfort is lessened, and often entirely absent.*

*As you begin labor, meditate on the tremendous universal force . . . the life force of nature with which you are in complete harmony during this experience.*

*Whenever you feel your body begin to surge, actively think "release" and "let go" of tension. There is a time for experiencing that uterine wave, flowing with it, and ultimately releasing and letting go.*

*You are learning to relax, to flow, and melt with the very rhythm of life itself. With relaxation and positive expectation, you have come to know that all things are possible.*

*In your mind's eye, picture the shore of a lake or an ocean. Watch the endless waves softly brushing to the shore . . . the ebb and flow of the water. Observe it advancing and withdrawing over the sand. Become a part of it, flowing into it. Become a part of the rhythm of the waves within your own body . . . the surge and release.*

*Breathe in the natural anesthesia of your own body . . . endorphins, many times more effective than the strongest drugs known to man . . . create your own serenity and release it throughout your body . . . breathing in and breathing through . . . giving birth to your baby.*

*With proper physical, spiritual, and mental exercise, you are preparing yourself for this wonderful celebration of life. As you get into the rhythm and work with your mind and body, the easier and smoother it becomes. Each time you hear your birth companion's voice and feel the gentle touch, the more easily your relaxation deepens.*

*Breathe . . . slowly, confidently, gently. Each time you breathe in, breathe in relaxation and peace. Each time you breathe out, breathe out stress, as the body's natural endorphins willfully breathe out tension and stress.*

*Feel only the sway of the wave that is bringing your baby closer and closer to birth. Relax and flow with your body's natural rhythm, confident in the fact that your body knows what to do. Give your birthing over to your body. Trust it. Relax and let it do its job.*

*With your mind's eye and your inner senses, mentally and emotionally feel yourself joyfully, totally aware, and participating. See it as already accomplished. Listen with your mind's ear to that first sound of new life.*

*Create a vivid visualization of the exhilaration you feel as you see your baby at the moment of birth. See the three of you bonding for the first time in this life. Now mentally see yourself stepping into this joyful scene. Become a part of this birthing . . . fulfilled. Feel it . . . Sense it. This is now your body. In your mind's eye, see and feel yourself totally enveloping that body . . . holding the baby on your breast. These are your arms enfolding your baby; these are your hands embracing this new little being.*

*You knew you could do it, and you did. You did well, and the feeling of ecstacy is one that will never be surpassed.*

*Join in with joy and amazement and watch the continuing mystery of creation unfold. The life force of nature is working in harmony with you. Now more than at any moment in your life, it is within you and with you. You are an integral part of nature, and nature is an integral part of your being. You are a part of the greatest celebration of life.*

*"You are a part of the promise and the destiny of life itself."*
Henry Leo Bolduc
<u>Self-Hypnosis - Creating Your Own Destiny</u>

# *Recommendations for Postnatal Bonding*

- As often as you can, hold the baby on the left near your heart. Babies need love and touching as much as they need nourishment.

- React to baby's communication (crying). Babies cry because something is upsetting or confusing to them as they attempt to adjust to their new existence outside of the womb.

- Make new affirmations and recite them during feeding or bathing. Talk and caress; you will love every minute of it.

- Repeat as many of the prenatal bonding experiences as possible so that the same familiar sounds and interactions can help the baby to adjust to its new life. Play your music tape to soothe fretful times.

- Refrain from any negative expression or tone toward the baby's bodily functions--stools, spitting up, burping.

- Avoid fatigue as much as possible and don't internalize the baby's "fretfulness." Don't do battle with this little being. He/she is not out to see that you never get a hot meal or a good night's rest. Remember, it isn't easy for baby, either. Stay calm.

- Avoid getting stressed. This is a good time to call back the techniques of relaxation that you've become an expert at. Listen to relaxation music as often as you can, even if you pause for only a few minutes at a time.

As hard as it may seem to believe at times, you will actually find that these first few months will go all too soon. You'll find yourself looking back on your baby's infancy and missing those wonderful moments when you and your baby were first getting acquainted. Very quickly the baby will pass through one stage after another; and before you know it, your baby will be a toddler. The attitude that you adopt during the early months will serve you well through these later challenges. On the previous page and below are some suggestions for that wonderful stage of growth and exploration when your child is discovering the world and its many wonders.

### *Please, Mom and Dad . . .*

*My hands are small. I don't mean to spill my milk.*

*My legs are short--Please slow down so I can keep up.*

*Don't slap my hands when I touch something bright and pretty. I don't understand.*

*Please look at me when I talk to you. It lets me know you are really listening.*

*My feelings are tender--don't nag me all day. Let me make mistakes without feeling stupid.*

*Don't expect the bed I make or the picture I draw to be perfect. Just love me for trying.*

*Remember, I am a child, not a small adult. Sometimes I don't understand what you're saying.*

*I love you so much. Please love me just for being myself, not just for the things I can do.*

-author unknown

# Relaxation And Breathing: The Keys to Success

Most athletes will readily advise that relaxation and visualization are crucial to successful performance. Golfers quickly learn not to "press," to release and let go. Sports greats know that stress and tension in the mind equate to stress and tension in the body; the two cannot be separated. Conquering stress and fear is what allows sports figures to appear to perform so effortlessly. It's impressive.

So, too, the serene look on the face of the HypnoBirthing mom as she experiences uterine surges is awe inspiring. Equally impressive is the smile that creeps onto her face as she alerts herself following a surge. There is no trace of exhaustion or dread as her gaze meets that of her birthing companion. The slow breathing and sleep breathing techniques learned in HypnoBirthing classes help her to be in touch with her own natural instincts--to let her body and her baby take over, while she experiences this wonderful event on a deeper level.

Taking the time to practice these techniques, therefore, becomes an essential part of your daily routine. Since you are conditioning your mind for ultimate relaxation, it is important that you form a pattern that your mind can automatically respond to when it comes time for your birthing. This is time well spent, and it can cut the time and the effort you will spend in your labor.

*"Muscles send messages to each other. Clenched fists, a tight mouth, a furrowed brow, all send signals to the birth-passage muscles, the very ones that need to be loosened. Opening up to relax these upper-body parts relaxes the lower ones."*

*Sears & Sears*
*The Birth Book*

# *Your Relaxation Program*

Proven to be one of the most effective tools for dealing with tension, stress, and discomfort without drugs is your own ability to slip into relaxation and visualization. In HypnoBirthing classes you will learn relaxation techniques and visualizations that will see you through your labor and also facilitate your rapid recovery following the birth of your baby. It is important that you rehearse these techniques so that you can call them up readily when they are needed in labor.

## ESTABLISHING YOUR ROUTINE

- Select a time to relax when you won't be disturbed. Take the phone off the hook.

- Set aside the same time each day and dedicate yourself to that time.

- Choose a practice spot that has soft, dim light; make that the place you will use daily.

- Be sure that your bladder is empty.

- Wear clothes that are not binding and use a soft throw over your body to ensure your being comfortably warm.

- Use HypnoBirthing tapes; the background music tape consists of tones that the body responds to best.

# *Positions for Relaxation*

Your own body will be the best source of information as to the position you will assume when doing relaxation with your tapes. The general rule of thumb is to use the position in which you feel most comfortable.

## BACK POSITION

• Early in your pregnancy, you will no doubt be comfortable on your back while you practice relaxation. Later in your pregnancy, you will want to elevate your head and shoulders a bit more to accommodate the extra weight of the baby. If you gain a considerable amount of weight, you may choose to use a different position. If you are lying flat, the pressure of the weight of your baby can block the main blood vessel in your back, the major vena cava, and shut off the supply of blood and oxygen to the lower part of your body and your baby.

• Let your arms rest at your sides; bend elbows slightly outward, with shoulders opening outward also.

• Hands should be gently and softly cupped, palms downward and fingers resting in a rounded position on a flat surface at your side.

• Feet should be about six inches apart, turned outward.

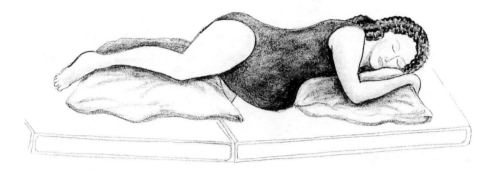

## LATERAL POSITION

The lateral position is a most important position, as it is the one chosen most frequently by birthing mothers during late labor and frequently for birthing. It is also a position that is frequently assumed for sleeping during the latter weeks of pregnancy.

- Lie on your left side with the left shoulder, neck, and left side of the head resting on a pillow. The left arm should be placed loosely by your left side.

- With the elbow bent, rest the right arm to the side of the pillow.

- The left leg should be straight down, with the knee slightly bent.

- Bend the right leg up, placing the knee even with your hip with one or two pillows under the knee for support.

## FACIAL RELAXATION

Achieving deep facial relaxation is most important, as it will set the tone for the rest of your body. When you have mastered the art of facial relaxation, your jaws will be totally relaxed, with the lower jaw slightly receded. You will be able to bring yourself into a natural state of relaxation instantly.

## TECHNIQUE

Let your eyelids slowly close. Don't try to force them shut. Just let them gently meet. Focus on the muscles in and around your eyes. As you feel a natural drooping of the eye muscles, sense relaxation spreading from your forehead, down across your eyelids, over your cheekbones, and around your jaws. Let your lower jaw recede as your teeth part. Your eyelids will feel heavier as your cheeks and your jaw go limp. Bring the relaxation within your eyes to a level where it will seem as though your eyelids just can't work. Feel your head making a dent into your pillow. As you practice this technique, you will feel your neck, your shoulders and your elbows droop. Picture your shoulders opening outward and your arms hanging limp from the elbow.

# *Breathing Techniques*

## SLEEP BREATHING

Oxygen is the most important fuel for the working muscles in the uterus. It is also important that your baby have a sufficient, continual supply of oxygen. That is why the proper breathing taught in HypnoBirthing is so important to your relaxation, and relaxation is so important to the success of your birthing. Sleep breathing, a slow, deep breathing, is the breathing technique you will use most frequently at the beginning of each relaxation practice. You will want to focus your attention on mastering this technique as early in your program as possible.

## TECHNIQUE

Sleep breathing will help you to achieve relaxation when you are practicing with your tapes or with your birth companion. It will also be the method you will use to resume relaxation between uterine surges during labor. It is this technique that will help you to conserve energy during the first stage of labor so that you will be able to maximize each breath during the second stage when you breathe your baby down to crowning. To establish a proper breathing technique for sleep breathing, practice the following exercise:

- Settle into a comfortable chair, recliner, or sofa; use one or two pillows to support your head and your neck. If sitting, allow your head to gently rest on your chest or let it rest back onto the pillows.

- For further comfort, roll or fold a pillow under your knees so hips, joints, and knees will be slightly bent.

• Let your eyelids gently meet; don't force them shut. Your mouth should be softly closed, with your lips barely touching.

• On the intake, draw your breath from your stomach. To a count of four, mentally recite, "In-2-3-4" on the intake. Feel your stomach rise as you draw the breath up and across your palate.

• As you exhale, mentally recite, "Out-2-3-4-5-6-7-8." Gently push your breath down through your throat and your chest, allowing your shoulders and your chest to droop inward into the frame of your body. Do not exhale through your mouth or directly through your nose. The push should be down and inward.

To check to see if you are doing this exercise correctly, place your left hand on your stomach and your right hand on the lower part of your chest. As you inhale, you should feel your left hand rising as though your stomach were inflating like a balloon. As you exhale, your right hand should sink into the cavity created by your drooping shoulders and chest.

Breathe your body down into relaxation, allowing your shoulders, elbows, and chest to droop into your torso more and more with each exhalation. "Release and let go."

Sleep breathing is easy to master. This is the breathing that you will use for practice sessions in your HypnoBirthing classes and for your home practice. You'll feel relaxation coming more easily and rapidly each time you do it, and you won't need to recite numbers to guide yourself into this state once you've mastered the technique.

## SLOW BREATHING

**SLOW BREATHING IS THE MOST IMPORTANT PART OF YOUR CHILDBIRTH PREPARATION.** Slow breathing is a <u>long</u>, quiet, slow intake of breath that redirects your focus to what is happening around your baby and helps you work with each surge. Slow breathing takes practice and MUST be worked on daily. A few minutes when you awaken in the morning and before you fall asleep at night should provide you ample practice.

When you first practice this breathing pattern, you will learn that its name is designed to indicate the manner of inspiration in which you are taking in <u>long, slow breaths</u>.

The goal of slow breathing is to make your breath, in and out, as long as possible to coincide with the length of the surge and to cause the abdominal wall to rise to as great a height as possible. This breathing helps you to maximize the efficiency of the surge. By working with the rise of the surge, you help the vertical muscles to draw up the lower circular fibers and open the cervix.

## TECHNIQUE

Lying on your back or in a lateral position, as described previously, place your hands across the top of your abdomen. Exhale briefly to clear your lungs and nasal passages. **Slowly** and gradually draw in your breath to a count from 1 to 20. **Avoid using short intakes of breath**; it can tire you and requires that you take several breaths in order to get through the surge. The intake count up to 20 and the equally slow exhalation will allow you sufficient time to work with each surge. If it is necessary for you to take a second breath during a surge, do so in the very same manner. Do not hold your breath--ever.

Keep your body still and limp--NOT STIFF--visualize your abdomen as being similar to a crater. The rest of your body beneath the crater is totally relaxed and still while you breathe up each surge. The Glove Relaxation technique that you will learn later is a good technique to use throughout this time when you will be working with your surges in the first stage.

While breathing in, focus your attention on your rising abdomen and bring the surge up as much as you can; visualize filling a balloon as you draw in. **Slowly** exhale to the same count, breathing downward and outward. Visualize the balloon slowly drifting off into space. Give your breath to your baby, gently and slowly exhaling down into your vagina.

You may find at first that you will reach an intake count of only 13 to 15. This is not unusual. You'll stretch the count more each time you do this exercise, and your count will rapidly increase to the long, slow intake. Regardless of how high a count you achieve, the technique of fully expanding the abdomen will be with you when you need it for labor. When each surge takes place, you will feel the results of your practice, as you successfully work with the surge in appropriately long intakes of breath and equally long exhalation. As when doing sleep breathing, you won't need to use the count once you have learned how to do the technique.

*"Imagine a magnificent, colored balloon. Each count of your breath brings more and more air into the balloon until, at last, the filled balloon gently drifts out over the landscape of your mind, and you slowly breathe down to prepare for the next balloon."*

# *Progressive Relaxation*

Once your breathing has become rhythmic and you can bring yourself into relaxation easily, you can deepen the relaxation rapidly by using progressive relaxation, illustrated below. Associate each part of your body from the top of your head to your toes with the corresponding number. Eventually, you will be able to take one deep breath, think the numbers as you exhale, and bring those parts of your body immediately into relaxation. The more rapidly you think the numbers, the more rapidly you will feel the effects.

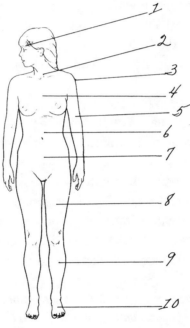

# *Disappearing Letters*

An excellent technique for bringing yourself into instant relaxation or deepening the level of your relaxation is to use the Disappearing Letters Exercise. It is perhaps the easiest of all that you will use.

## TECHNIQUE

• Close your eyes

• Take a deep breath -- Pause

• Quickly and quietly say to yourself while you exhale:

### AAA - BBB - CCC - D

• Allow your shoulders and your upper torso to just sink into the frame of your body.

With practice, you will find that by the time you reach the first D, the rest of the letters of the alphabet will be erased from your mind. This exercise is one of the fastest ways to bring yourself into a wonderful state of deep relaxation.

# *Hypnotic Analgesia and Visualizations*

## *Rainbow Relaxation*

The "Rainbow Relaxation" is the script for the reading that is on the HypnoBirthing relaxation tape. The background music is a composition by Steven Halpern, world-renowned author, composer and recording artist, whose sounds are designed to bring your thoughts into harmony with the natural flow of energy within the body. We have been using this piece, except for a very brief period of time, since the inception of HypnoBirthing. When we compared the results of the period when we weren't using this tape with the results that we had before and after, we found that there is, indeed, a difference in the ease with which our mothers give birth when using this particular music tape. We enthusiastically suggest that this music is conducive to bringing a laboring mother into a beautifully relaxed state, creating a peaceful birthing environment. (Steven Halpern's music tape is available through your Practitioner or from the HypnoBirthing Institute.)

You should use the entire HypnoBirthing Rainbow Relaxation tape for your own practice daily. Your practice with your birthing companion can be limited to the reading of only two or three colors of the rainbow script that will be provided to you by your HypnoBirthing Practitioner. You can alternate the rainbow with "A Father's Script" that is in your text. The practice that you do together is intended to strengthen the conditioning that comes from your learning to respond to your birth companion's voice. Using only two or three colors or the shorter Father's Script for each practice will prevent your practice from becoming a lengthy chore that can be put off until you can "find more time."

## TECHNIQUE

Once you have brought yourself into a state of relaxation, picture yourself resting on a bed of strawberry-colored mist that is about a foot and a half high. Picture the soft red mist as a mist of natural relaxation flowing around your body. Continue relaxing until it seems that your body is almost weightless and seems to meld into the mist. Feel the colored mist caressing your shoulders, your buttocks, and your legs. <u>Allow</u> yourself to "let go" and feel as though you are floating on the strawberry-colored mist. Feel the gentle sway. See this soft mist penetrating your body as you go deeper into relaxation. Feel your body growing numb, almost as though it were a lifeless piece of soft, strawberry-colored cloth--no feeling. Allow yourself to feel the mist of deep relaxation permeating your mind and body, causing a total sense of weightlessness. See your own natural endorphins swirling over and around your body--mind and body at peace and tranquil.

Now picture yourself resting on a bed of pale, orange-colored mist while your body becomes more and more weightless. Follow the same visualization as you did for the soft red. Continue the visualization until you have sequentially pictured yourself on all of the remaining colors of the rainbow--yellow, green, blue, indigo, and violet. Each visualization will cause you to become more profoundly relaxed. You may even experience a swaying sensation. This technique and imagery is important, as it will be used by the birth companion along with the Glove Relaxation technique (Page 83) during your birthing. These are the kinds of suggestions that will facilitate the flow of natural endorphins throughout your body while you are in the first stage of labor. You will use the mist of the rainbow to spread the body's natural anesthesia whenever a surge comes on. Go only with your breathing and your visualization, not your body. Let your body continue to lie limp and numb.

As often as possible, the birth companion should practice with you, stroking your hand and arm in an upward motion, simulating the flow of anesthesia from the glove of relaxation. Whether this practice is done with or without the birth companion, it is one of the most important. **Use it daily**.

I often hear that after only a few practice sessions, mothers slip into a deep relaxation even before they get to the colors. If you find that this is true for you, you're well on your way to easier birthing.

The Father's Script is a good reading that you and your companion can use to vary your practice together. Visualizing yourself stepping into the scene is important for creating an imprint of a positive outcome.

# *The Opening Blossom*

One of the most effective visualizations for use during second-stage labor is that of an opening rose. As you envision your baby moving gently into the vaginal opening, imagine that opening to be like a rose bud. See the petals of the rose slowly and easily unfolding and opening to allow the baby to slip out. The perineal massage that you do during the last six to eight weeks of your pregnancy will give you the confidence to see this happening.

It is believed that the pressure of the descending head creates its own anesthesia, just as other parts of your body become numb when there is pressure applied to them. As soon as the perineum is fully stretched, it loses sensation and becomes quite anesthetized. Follow your opening rose visualization and feel the outlet stretching and the numbing effect that the pressure has on the entire region.

# *Blue Satin Ribbons*

While you are in a surge, the vertical muscles of your uterus draw the lower circular muscles fibers up and back to effect the dilation of your cervix. In between surges, visualize these lower fibers as being soft, blue satin ribbons that gently and easily yield to the rhythmic draw of the vertical muscles, swirling up and back, allowing the neck of the cervix to open.

# *Arm-Wrist Relaxation Test*

Because you don't really experience a particular sensation when you are in self-hypnosis, you will be amused and amazed at the arm-wrist relaxation test. It is very simple and, at the same time, very convincing. The technique is reassuring to both the birth companion and the mother-to-be.

## TECHNIQUE

The arm-wrist relaxation test is most effectively practiced by lying on your back, with your arms at your side, your fingers gently cupped on the surface of the bed or sofa. Do not lie flat on your back for long periods of time when you are in the late stages of pregnancy or in labor.

Once you are in a state of relaxation, picture that your birth companion has tied a giant, red, helium-filled balloon to your right wrist. Almost immediately you will begin to feel a tug on your wrist as the balloon pulls upward. Now add another helium-filled balloon--this time orange. The two balloons are tugging even harder on your wrist. Your arm is beginning to rise upward. With each tug, your arm is being pulled higher. Still another balloon--a yellow one--is being added. Each time a balloon is added, your arm begins to feel lighter and lighter. The more you try to hold your wrist down, the more the helium is pulling your arm upward. Continue to picture more balloons being added.

Your arm now cannot resist the pull of the balloons. Though you try to hold it down, your wrist is being yanked upward. The tug on your wrist is stronger. Your arm is rising in spite of your efforts to hold it down.

When your arm rises approximately six to ten inches off the bed, place it back at your side. Each time you practice this exercise, fewer balloons will be required to make your arm and wrist tilt upward. At the end of each relaxation period, tell yourself that each time you practice, relaxation will take over your body sooner than ever before.

Your goal should be to assume a deep level of relaxation within a very short period of time. Become familiar with each of these techniques so that you can vary them when you are in labor. Practice alerting yourself, returning to instant relaxation, and alerting yourself again. You will want to be able to do this when you experience a uterine surge during labor.

# *The Depthometer*

A technique that has been found to be extremely effective in deepening relaxation to a point where the body is almost totally limp is a variation on "Yardstick Imagery."

## TECHNIQUE

The method involves visualizing a large, flexible, inverted thermometer, placed inside your body with the bulb above your forehead, and the flexible tube extending all the way down to your toes. Inside the bulb is a silvery fluid of numbing relaxation. There are 40 gradations on the thermometer. As you count down from 40 to 39 to 38, etc., picture the fluid of relaxation gently flowing down from one number to the next. To reinforce the concept of relaxation filling your body, visualize more natural endorphins in the silvery fluid of relaxation flowing down into the tube of the thermometer. You will feel a deep relaxation gradually saturating your body as the fluid fills the space in the tube. As you slowly count down, at the end of each decade, the numbers--30, 20, 10--will bring you to a new and deeper level. By the time you reach the lower teens, you will find yourself in a very deep relaxation. The final decade will bring you to the deep relaxation you will use during the latter part of the first stage of labor.

This is an imagery that you can use alone or with your birthing companion. Your birthing companion can recite this imagery to you during labor.

## The Sensory Gate Valve

This is a very simple imagery that, like Glove Anesthesia, helps to bring about a loss of sensation in selected parts of the body. The imagery puts you into the control center of the inner mind, where you see yourself adjusting the dial on the face of a large round valve that disconnects any message from the mind concerning pain. When the dial is moved to the "OFF" position, the concept of pain cannot pass through the sensory gate in the stem of the brain. In HypnoBirthing classes, a hypnotic induction is practiced that brings you in imagery to the control center of your mind. Here, you learn to deactivate any part of your body where you want to deflect feelings of discomfort. The following script can be used by a birthing companion or you can create your own tape. The important thing is that your body becomes conditioned to shut off messages of discomfort that could come through the sensory gate. This exercise demonstrates how the technique works, as you practice numbing a hand and a foot.

## TECHNIQUE

Imagine yourself at the control center of your inner mind; see in front of you a large valve with three settings on the face of the valve. At the center of the top of the valve is the normal position, "ON." When the indicator is positioned at this setting, you are able to move any part of your body, and you would feel pain if you were to injure yourself. You will see yourself able to move and function normally. With practice, when the indicator is mentally switched to the "OFF" position, which is approximately at the eight o'clock position on the face of a clock, your entire body becomes numb and immobile. You will be able to feel pressure and movement within your uterus, but the rest of your body will feel numb and senseless, and unresponsive.

Now if you mentally switch the indicator to the SELECT position-- at approximately the four o'clock position on the valve--you will be able to move any part of your body, but you will not be able to move your right hand and you cannot lift your right foot. Try as you may, you will not be able to lift your right foot or move your right hand. It's as though your hand is stuck to your lap and your foot is glued to the floor. Go ahead, try. to move your right hand or foot. You cannot. Your right hand and foot are numb. But now you can move the fingers of your left hand and lift your left foot. Do it. See how easily they move.

Now put the indicator back to the normal position of "ON" and lift your right hand and your right foot. All mobility has returned.

During labor you may elect to leave just the abdominal or pelvic parts of your body in a numbed, analgesic state by selecting the "SELECT" position, or you can numb your entire body by visualizing the dial on the control valve at the "OFF" position.

*HypnoBirthing*
*Control Valve*

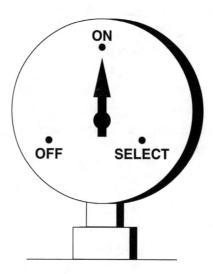

*". . . The partner's encouragement and practical help increase the effectiveness of labor-coping techniques, such as creative imagery and breathing patterns. The presence also increases the woman's chance of an emotionally fulfilling birth."*

*Carl Jones*
*The Birth Partner's Handbook*

# Glove Relaxation

Imagine that you are putting a soft, silver glove onto your right hand--a special glove of natural endorphins. Immediately you can feel the fingers of your hand begin to tingle, as though there were springs at the ends of your fingers. The silver glove, with its endorphins flowing around your fingers, your palm, and the back of your hand, will cause your hand to feel numb, the way it would if you were to place it into a large container of icy slush. The visualization helps to release the body's endorphins.

## TECHNIQUE:

As your birth companion strokes the back of your hand and arm, feel a tingling and then a numbness surrounding your hand and moving up your arm. Once your hand and your arm lose all sensation, they begin to seem as lifeless and senseless as a piece of wood or a piece of leather. The silver mist of numbness gradually drifts throughout your body wherever you transfer it. To transfer the numbing effect, just visualize placing your hand on various parts of your body--each part now feels light, numb, and senseless. Use the colors of the mist of the rainbow to spread this natural calm throughout your body whenever a uterine surge comes on.

Practice will condition your body to react with calm when you feel your hand and arm being stroked. Go only with your breathing, and your visualizations, not your body. Let your body continue to lie totally limp and senseless. Even moms who claim to feel uncomfortable with the stroking practice fall into relaxation during labor and ask that the companion use stroking while giving relaxation prompts.

# Light Touch Massage

In HypnoBirthing classes, birthing companions are taught the art of Light Touch Massage, a technique developed by Constance Palinsky after much research into pain management and relaxation methods. The technique is very simple, yet very effective. It is a wonderful comfort measure that the birthing companion brings to the labor room.

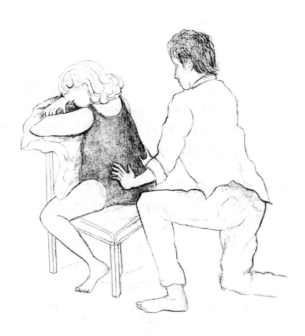

**BIRTH COMPANION PREPARES TO APPLY LIGHT TOUCH**

Just below the surface of the skin, attached to the hair follicles, is a smooth muscle called the erector pili. This muscle reacts to stimuli by contracting. When this occurs, the muscle pulls up the surface hair, becomes erect, and causes goose bumps. The goose bumps, in turn, help to create endorphins, enabling you to relax.

Light Touch Massage can be applied during labor if you choose to change to a kneeling position as an alternative labor position.

In setting up for Light Touch Massage in a hospital, the birthing companion can request that the foot of the hospital bed be adjusted to create a kneeler. With your knees on a pillow on the kneeler and your arms supported by pillows that have been stacked upright on the end or side of the bed, you can continue to relax during surges. This position also enables you to utilize the pull of gravity, even though you are not totally erect. The same effect can be achieved by kneeling on a pillow in front of a chair, a sofa, or at the side of a bed with pillows stacked upright for you to rest your arms and head on. Your birthing companion can kneel behind you while administering Light Touch Massage. You will receive an extra bonus if your companion uses light touch while you are sitting at your bedside with your legs spread on the top of a birthing ball.

## TECHNIQUE

The birthing companion places his/her hands at the small of the back to become centered. Using the <u>back</u> side of the fingers, the companion places his/her hands so that they meet at the base of the spine. The fingers are then drawn up and out from the spine in a V-like motion. The pattern is gradually continued upward across the back until the base of the neck is reached. The hands are then brought around the neck and to the sides of the ears.

The second motion involves placing the back of the fingers at the base of the spine and then, as before, gradually working upward, forming a horizontal, figure-eight pattern that criss crosses at the center of the back.

Normally, when light touch is applied in a massage setting, the practitioner is cautioned not to extend the hands near the breasts or ears, as these are erogenous zones. Just the opposite is true during labor. If the birthing companion extends his hands out and around the sides of the breasts and nipples, not only are endorphins produced, but also a hormone--oxytocin--is created that naturally enhances uterine surges.

Your HypnoBirthing practitioner will provide you with specific instructions and diagrams for using Light Touch Massage.

## *Time Distortion*

Once you have mastered the art of bringing yourself into relaxation easily, you may want to begin practicing time distortion. When you are in a relaxed state, give yourself the suggestion that every five minutes will seem as one minute. When you are in the mid-to-late first stage of labor, the birthing companion will give you the suggestion that every twenty minutes will seem as five. Time distortion is an important part of birthing and is included among the prompts that the birth companion uses. Along with an amnesiac state that occurs toward the end of the first stage of labor, time distortion is indeed a gift that nature bestows on the laboring mother.

# *Preparing Your Body for Birthing*

## *Body Exercises*

It is particularly important for you to exercise during pregnancy. It is also important, however, that you don't build exercising into a routine that becomes an ordeal or a time-consuming chore. You will want to find ways to tone your body that are as natural as the birthing you are preparing for. Vary the exercises that you do and create a habit of doing them as often as you can as you go about your day-to-day activities. You'll discover that many of the exercises can be practiced incidentally. Some can even be done right on your bed as you awaken in the morning or just before you settle in to go to sleep at night.

## WALKING

Walking is one of the best exercises you can engage in. It helps to strengthen your breathing, as well as your legs. You don't have to follow a strict regimen of walking, but you can look for ways in which you can get in a little extra walking time; for example, park a distance from the entrance to your work or from the supermarket. Use an entrance that is not immediately adjacent to your destination. Rather than calling or taking an elevator to another area, find occasions to walk within the building at work. Walk as often as you can.

## AVOIDING BACK STRAIN

As your pregnancy advances, you will want to alleviate back strain by being aware of correct posture. Pregnant or not, a good assist to proper posture is to envision a string, passing from a point in front of the ear, down through the shoulders and the hipbone to a spot just behind the ankle bone. Keeping your head in line with this imaginary string will prevent you from "leading with your head," will keep your pelvis tilted back, and will help you to avoid stooping as you gain in weight and size. Don't lean back with your head behind the imaginary line; it will cause you to project your abdomen forward and will lead to the "pregnancy waddle." Many women assume this posture, with toes turned outward, long before final "dropping" has occurred.

Another exercise that is helpful in relieving back strain is the "pelvic rock." This exercise helps to avoid back strain, strengthens abdominal muscles, and increases the flexibility of your lower back. There are several ways to do the pelvic rock. Instructions for two methods follow on the next page.

**First Method:** Using a table-height, sturdy chair or other piece of furniture for arm support and balance, stand approximately two feet from the object. Bend your knees very slightly. Lean forward from your hips and thrust your buttocks backward. Allow your abdominal muscles to relax, creating a sway back. Bend your knees a little more and pull your hips forward, tucking your buttocks under as though you were being shooed from behind with a broom. Repeat the procedure several times.

**Second Method:** You can also practice the pelvic rock in a lying position during the early weeks of your pregnancy. On your back with your knees bent and your feet flat on the floor, tighten your lower abdominal muscles and the muscles of your buttocks. Your tailbone will rise, pressing the small of your back to the floor. Hold this position for a few seconds and then release the muscles. As you do this exercise, arch your back as much as you can. Repeat the procedure several times. You will also find this an excellent technique for flattening the abdomen following birthing.


## STRETCHING THE INNER THIGH AND LEG MUSCLES

At the end of the second stage of labor when you are breathing your baby down out of the birth canal and into the world, you may be in positions with your knees turned outward or raised upward. Understanding this, you know that THE INNER THIGH MUSCLES NEED TO BE STRETCHED.


* In stretching inner thigh muscles, the best effect can be derived from sitting on the floor or a bed with the soles of your feet together. Lean slightly forward and place your hands <u>on your ankles.</u> With your elbows resting on the end of your knees, gently press your elbows onto

your knees. As you do this exercise over time, gradually and gently pull your heels toward your crotch until your heels and your crotch meet and your knees almost rest on the floor. Once you have achieved this muscle tone, you should straighten your back during subsequent practice sessions.

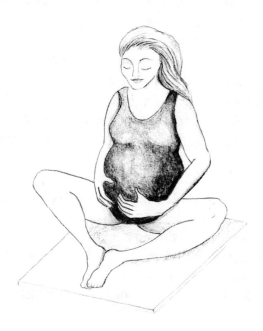

**Stretching Inner Thigh Muscles**

- Using the same technique as described previously, have your birth companion assist by placing his or her hands under your knees to create resistance. Press your elbows down upon your knees while your birth companion resists.

- In a semi-sitting position with your knees bent and raised upward toward your shoulders, place the palms of your hands against the under part of your knees and pull your knees outward. Bring your knees together again and then pull them apart. It is important that you do this to strengthen your legs. Do this about five to six times in each practice session.

- Squatting, rather than bending, is the way in which you should reach for low objects or lift an object or a small child. Do not attempt to lift heavy objects. In addition to facilitating your ability to lift objects, squatting is an excellent way to stretch the muscles of the inner thighs.

- Using a piece of furniture for balance, squat down onto your toes or feet and spread your knees outward. Using your leg muscles, slowly rise. Practice this several times a day. This exercise will tone and strengthen your leg muscles also.


## THE LEAPING FROG STRETCH

The leaping frog position comes to us from our practitioners in the Virgin Islands. Squatting is a position that is used throughout much of the world, though not as yet widely accepted in the United States. Not only does this position help to tone your muscles, but it also provides you with one of the best positions to labor during the second stage. While women in other cultures regularly use a squatting position for birthing, it must be remembered that these women use this posture for much of what they do on a daily basis. Western women are not naturally inclined to squatting, so this posture needs practice. The time that you spend in practicing this modified form of squatting will be well spent.

Assuming the leaping frog position during labor offers benefits for both you and your baby when you are breathing down or pushing. Just a few of the benefits of the leaping frog are:

- Widens the pelvic opening
- Relaxes and opens the perineal muscles
- Helps to avoid tearing and lessens the need for an episiotomy
- Relieves strain in the lower back
- Increases the supply of oxygen to your baby
- Shortens the birth canal
- Allows you a clear view of your baby's birth
- Makes better use of the effect of gravity

Though I recommend the leaping frog positions, to attempt to adopt these positions for any length of time when your muscles are not adequately toned could result in pain or injury to your leg muscles.

## TECHNIQUE

When first practicing the leaping frog position, you may need some help in the way of support to get down into the proper position. Your birthing companion can help by standing behind you so that you can lean your back against his legs, while he holds your hands for balance. The companion can also stand in front of you to assist you as you slowly lower your body down into position.

From a standing position with your feet spread about a foot and a half apart, assume a squatting position on your toes with your knees spread outward. Place your hands on the floor on either the inside or the outside of your legs.

As you continue to practice and squat rather than bend to reach for something that is low, your muscles will become toned. Gradually, you will be able to place your feet flat on the floor as the muscles at the back of your legs and heels become toned.

A variation of this position is to assume a kneeling position with your legs spread wide and to the side. Lower your body onto your legs, with your buttocks resting on your heels. Place your hands in front of you. This position can be converted into an all-fours stance, by simply moving your hands farther front and raising your body from your buttocks.

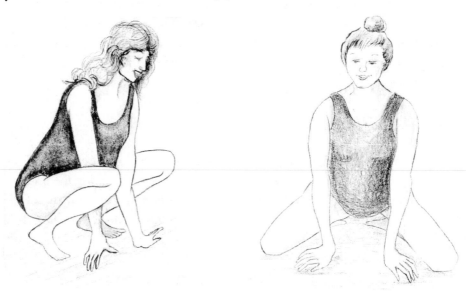

**Leaping Frog Positions**

# Kegel Exercises

These exercises, named for the Austrian doctor who first recommended their use, are also known as pelvic floor exercises. Not enough attention is paid to Kegels. They are among the most important of all the prenatal muscle toning. Designed to tone and strengthen the muscles used during the second stage of birthing, these exercises involve the muscles that form a figure eight around the vaginal and anal region. As illustrated in the drawing that follows, the muscles create a network that surrounds the entire pelvic area. Kegels also serve the very important function of restoring the stretched and dilated openings to their normal size after labor and are helpful in preventing some of the urinary problems connected with aging. Control of this area can actually enhance lovemaking after having a child and avoid the all-too-common and unnecessary complaint of uninteresting sex because of stretched, relaxed muscles. You will enjoy the confidence derived from well-toned anal and vaginal sphincters as your pregnancy advances and there is more pressure on the bladder and bowel.

## TECHNIQUE

In a sitting position, start by contracting the lowest muscles of the anal and vaginal tracts as tightly as you can. Keep tightening the muscles until you can feel the contracted muscles all the way up into the top of the vagina and you get the sensation of pulling the anus into the rectum. It is helpful to count from one to ten as you do these exercises, tightening a little more with each number. When you have tightened all of the muscles, hold the contraction for a few seconds and then release slowly.

These muscles are the same ones used to stop the flow of urine. To see if you are doing this exercise correctly, try to stop the flow of urine while you are urinating. Do not attempt to stop the flow of urine once you have established that you are doing the exercise correctly; to do this more than is necessary could result in a urinary tract infection. Be sure to practice this exercise several times a day, doing the exercise 5 to 6 times at each practice. Frequent practice is all to your benefit. The exercises can be done easily at any time, anywhere, whether at work or at home. The important thing is-- DO IT.

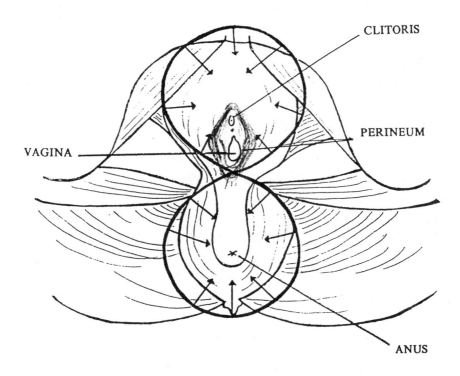

**The network of muscles surrounding the pelvic floor**

# Perineal Massage

Perineal Massage is one of the oldest and surest ways of improving the health, blood flow, elasticity, and relaxation of the pelvic floor muscles. Practiced in late pregnancy, this technique improves the chances of birthing your baby without an episiotomy. <u>The importance of this massage cannot be overemphasized.</u> When your perineal rim is soft and relaxed, your baby easily slips past the rim and out of the vagina. It is far better for you to stretch these tissues beforehand than to have your medical caregiver do it while you are crowning. Attention to this massage will pay off. It is simple and yet so effective. YOU WILL WANT TO TAKE IT SERIOUSLY.

Massaging with oil helps to stretch the perineal muscles and soften the tissue, both of which will reduce resistance to the baby's head. As you or your partner do the massage, you can learn to identify which muscles you will need to relax in childbirth; and you can teach these muscles to relax and open outward in response to pressure.

The massage should be done **every day for at least five minutes**, beginning about six to eight weeks before your due date. Because of your increased size and the awkwardness of bending around your abdomen, it may be easier to have someone else do the massage for you. If you are doing the massage by yourself you'll find it easier if you place one foot on the seat of a chair, with the other approximately two or three feet away from the chair. This allows you to work around and under your abdomen.

Be sure that fingernails are smooth and short when doing the massage. A rubber glove will ensure that there are no rough surfaces to irritate the vaginal tissue. You may use virgin olive oil, sweet oil, almond oil, baby oil, or a lubricating gel. Avoid perfumed oils.

## TECHNIQUE

Pour a little of the oil into a custard cup or shallow bowl. (Be sure to discard oil that is left after massaging.)

Sit with your back resting against pillows and get comfortable. It's a good idea to use a mirror during the first few times that you do this exercise. It will assist you in identifying the muscles that are involved and will allow you to observe the stretching of the edge of the perineum.

Dip your thumb into the oil and thoroughly moisten it. If a partner is doing the massage, he will use his first and middle fingers. The thumb or fingers should be dipped into the oil to the second knuckle and inserted into the vagina approximately 2-3", pressing downward on the area between the vagina and the rectum. Rub the oil into the inner edge of the perineum and the lower vaginal wall.

Maintaining a steady pressure, slide the fingers upward along the sides of the vagina in a "U," sling-type motion. This pressure will stretch the vaginal tissue, the muscles surrounding the vagina, and the outer rim of the perineum. Be sure to stretch the inner portions, as well as the outer rim of the perineum. In the beginning you will feel the tightness of the muscles; but with time and practice, the tissue will relax.

Practice relaxing the extended muscles by picturing the perineum opening outward as pressure is applied. The opening rosebud is a good visualization to use during this exercise.

---

# Getting Ready to
# Welcome Your Baby

---

## Setting the Stage

So far you've been doing all of the right things in preparing yourself mentally and physically for your baby's birth. Now, as the days wind down, it's time to start tying the ends together.

The best way to help ensure that your birth experience is positive, healthy, and safe for you and your baby is to thoroughly prepare and plan. Sitting down together and deciding what is important to you will certainly increase the chances of your being able to experience that most satisfying birth that you are seeking.

# *Your Birth Plan*

Too often couples come away from their birthing experiences expressing their disappointment with phrases such as, "Oh well, the next time . . ." or, "If only they hadn't . . . ."

If you and your birthing companion have a clear vision of what will allow you to have the most natural, gentle, and satisfying birthing for you and your baby, you'll not find yourselves looking on as your birthing is controlled by others.

In the absence of having your plan in hand, medical staff will follow their usual and routine procedures, assuming that you have prepared for your birthing through childbirth classes that are not as parent and baby oriented as HypnoBirthing is. Most nurses in the labor and birthing area are there because they feel a strong dedication to being part of the birthing miracle and are more than willing to assist you in making your birthing the special event that you have planned.

To ensure that your birthing does not needlessly turn into a "medical incident," you will need to select medical caregivers who will listen to you and respect your philosophy and your wishes. Talking with your doctor or midwife should take place early in your pregnancy and not simply be left to a chance conversation later on.

If you've selected a clinic or association that has a rotating staff of physicians, any one of whom could be attending your birth, make several copies and ask that each medical attendant be given a copy of your Birth Plan.

If you plan to have a home birth, you will want to see that your midwife, and anyone else who will be present, has a copy of the plan. Guests should know that you have a plan in place and this is not the time to relate stories of the progress of their own labors or attempt to give you advice. You are the stars, directors, and producers in this play.

In framing your plan, keep in mind that your intent is not to "take on" your medical caregivers or practices that are currently in effect in the hospital or center. Word your plan in such a way that it does not become an adversarial document of demands. You will also want to assure your medical providers that they will have your full cooperation should a medical necessity arise.

A copy of a suggested outline for a Birth Plan appears at the end of this book. Your HypnoBirthing instructor will give you a worksheet copy for your own use, along with a letter to your health care provider. Depending upon where you live, some of the choices on the plan may not apply. You may skip any items that you do not feel strongly about one way or the other. There is room on the plan after each section to put additional requests or comments.

## *Hospital or Birthing Center Visit*

Your HypnoBirthing classes provide you with information and techniques that help you develop confidence as you approach your birthing. To add another measure of confidence, it is helpful for you and your birthing companion to visit the hospital or birthing center sometime in advance of your anticipated birthing. Getting these "housekeeping duties" out of the way will ensure that you will not get bogged down with unnecessary delays at the time of your admission. Take advantage of the opportunity to talk with staff and complete paperwork. Inform the staff that you are planning a relaxed birthing with HypnoBirthing and ask that it be noted in your file. Be sure to leave a copy of your Birth Plan and request that it be added to your records. If this is a first HypnoBirthing at this facility, take the time to explain a little about the method.

Use this visit to become familiar with the layout and environment of the center. Inquire about entrances that should be used in the event you arrive before or after the hours that the hospital or center is normally open to the public. Know where elevators and receiving desks are located. You don't want to find yourselves wandering around, lost, at a time when you should be "settling in" to your own room.

It's helpful to have an idea of the time it takes to travel to the center. Do a couple of "dry runs"--one during a heavily trafficked time of day and one on a Sunday or late evening. Check out alternative routes that may not be as heavily traveled as the one you usually take.

*"Do be positive. Convey two messages: First, this is a well-researched baby, and you are a prepared and informed parent. You are doing everything you can do to take care of your health and the health of your baby. Second, you are asking your caregivers to do likewise."*

*William & Martha Sears*
*The Birth Book*

# *When Baby is Breech*

In preparation for birthing, sometime during the latter part of pregnancy--around the 32nd to the 37th week--the baby rotates from the upright position in which he has spent most of his time in the uterus to a vertex position. In the vertex position the baby's head is properly positioned down at the mouth of the cervix. Because the head contains the brain and the skull, it is the heaviest part of the baby's body. Once the baby is almost fully developed, the natural pull of gravity is usually sufficient to draw the head down.

Most of the time this turning goes without any particular note, especially if it occurs while the mother is sleeping. The process can be thwarted, however, when the mother is experiencing fear or tension that results in a tight cervix. When this happens, the baby, deprived of an adequate amount of space in which to turn, is unable to complete the rotation and remains in the original, upright position. The baby's buttocks remain at the neck of the uterus in what is called "breech presentation." Sometimes the baby completes only a partial rotation, leaving a shoulder, an arm, or one or both feet positioned at the lower part of the cervix.

A breech position, if not reversed, poses difficulty and risk. The options are limited to making every effort to help the baby turn, to deliver in the breech position, or to resort to a surgical delivery.

## HELPING THE BREECH-POSITIONED BABY TO TURN

HypnoBirthing techniques have proven very effective in helping the breech-presented baby to spontaneously reposition into vertex position on its own. This concept is buttressed in a study, presented in May of 1992, by Dr. Lewis Mehl, formerly of the Psychiatric Department, University of Vermont Medical School. The study included 100 women who were referred from practicing obstetricians and an additional 100 who responded to advertisement. Only women who were found to be carrying their babies in breech position at 36 weeks gestation or more were included. Dr. Mehl approached this study looking at reports on serial ultrasound examinations and abdominal palpation that suggested that the likelihood of a breech-positioned baby turning after the 37th week was no more than 12%.

Mehl used hypnotherapy with the 100 women in the study group. The comparison group of 100 women had no hypnotherapy, though some did have ECV (external cephalic version), a procedure whereby the baby's head is manually manipulated from outside the abdomen to bring about the downward turn.

In the study group the mothers, while in hypnosis, were led through guided imagery to bring about deep relaxation. Suggestions were then given that they visualize their babies easily turning and see the turn accomplished, with the baby in proper vertex position for birthing. The mothers were helped to visualize the uterus becoming pliable and relaxed in order to allow the baby sufficient room to make the move. The mother was asked to talk to her baby, and the therapist encouraged the baby to release itself from the position it had settled into and to turn downward for an easy birth.

The study ended in 1992, with the significant result that 81 of the 100 breech babies in the study group turned spontaneously from breech position to vertex position. It was originally thought that each mother would require approximately ten hours of hypnotherapy in order to accomplish the desired result. As the study unfolded, the average number of hours spent with each woman was only four; and half of the successful 81 turns required only one session.

In the comparison group of 100 women who did not participate in hypnotherapy, only 26 babies turned spontaneously. An additional 20 turned with ECV. It should be noted that it is not uncommon for the baby who is turned through ECV to turn back into breech position. The figures arrived at through this study are considered medically quite significant.

While there are no published data available on the relationship between the emotional state of the mother and the fetal position, there is literature showing that a presence of negative emotions or maternal anxiety and stress can have an adverse effect on the fetus and the new born baby.

A summary of this literature suggests that there is a definite relationship between maternal anxiety and the need for oxytocin initiation of labor. The study also indicates a more frequent use of labor drugs and augmentation, as well as the occurrence of fetal distress and cesarean section births.

From these findings we see that, in addition to working with visualization conducive to relaxing the uterus, mothers with babies in breech position can be helped through release therapy. Anxious moms need to let go of fears concerning their pregnancy, birthing, or parenting, and emotions from past experiences that could have a bearing on their tension and fear. Release therapy is an integral part of the HypnoBirthing Program, where mothers are helped to identify and release negative emotions. If your baby is in breech presentation, seek the assistance of your HypnoBirthing Practitioner; inquire about "tilting" exercises; and then consider ECV (external cephalic version) if it is still necessary. ECV should be a last resort. It is not usually a procedure of choice.

I have had the thrill of successfully using this therapy to turn breech presented babies. The first couple, Donna and Denny B., called to express their disappointment at having learned that their baby was in breech position. The prospects for cesarean birth hung heavily over the excitement that they had been feeling about their upcoming birthing. They were extremely excited about the HypnoBirthing method, and now they felt let down. They remembered that I had talked about Dr. Mehl's study and Dr. Andrew Weil's account of his wife Sabine's experience of having her posterior-positioned baby turn as a result of hypnosis. Donna and Denny asked for help.

I was disappointed at hearing their news, but I was also optimistic that if we were able to get Donna's uterus relaxed and help her and the baby bring about this needed turn, the cesarean could be avoided. Donna couldn't understand how this could be happening to her because she had totally embraced the HypnoBirthing philosophy and was not aware of feeling fearful. A telephone call while I was at her home gave a clue. Donna and Denny were in the throes of closing on a home that had a flawed deed. The heirs of the previous owners, though the property was no longer in the family, were refusing to sign off on the deed unless they were paid additional money. The bantering had gone on for weeks. The frustration and quiet anger that Donna was feeling was very evident in her voice, on her face, and, of course, in her cervix.

I met with Donna for a hypnotic session only once. We worked on release therapy and on visualization for a smooth and easy turn for the baby. We both talked to the baby, and I left her a tape that reinforced these suggestions.

When I answered the phone a couple of days later, Donna was on the other end of the line. When I heard her news, I was as ecstatic as she.

The baby had indeed turned. Donna was not aware of when the turn took place, but her doctor confirmed that the baby was in perfect position for birthing and that the head was, in fact, quite low. Two days later, after a wonderful labor in which Donna says she felt no uterine pain, a beautiful baby boy was born.

Donna's circumstances were even more remarkable because she had undergone three back fusions and was in constant pain as a result of an accident several years prior. With the relaxation and imagery that she practiced daily, Donna's back pain was eased. Her doctor commented that he doubted that she could have had her baby vaginally had it not been for her HypnoBirthing training. Donna's baby, incidentally, was born one month and one day ahead of the estimated due date. The baby was a fully developed 6 lb. 7 oz. boy. Here we see the merits of placing only a limited amount of emphasis on an exact "due date."

# Before Labor

## When The Baby Is Ready

There is a biblical reference to a woman's sorrowing that her time to birth has come. I've not done studies on it and have no statistics to support my belief; but from working with HypnoBirthing mothers, my experience tells me that our mothers welcome the early signs. These are indications that Nature is playing its part in tuning up for the main concert.

Sometime around nine-plus months from the time of the last menstrual period, the baby will begin to give signals that it is ready to be born. The uterus is "ripe," and labor begins. It is believed that a hormone secreted from within the baby's body triggers oxytocin, the natural labor-initiating hormone within the mother's body, and the miracle unfolds.

## EARLY SIGNALS

**Braxton-Hicks:** Much talked about, but little understood, Braxton-Hicks contractions are Nature's way of preparing the uterus for your baby's birthing. Named for the doctor who first defined these uterine surges, the contractions are much like the tightening sensations that are felt during labor. For first babies, these tightening surges will probably show up sometime during the end of the seventh month. For subsequent pregnancies, they may appear as early as the sixth month. Interestingly enough, Braxton-Hicks will sometimes give you a jolt with their pressurelike waves, but they are not accompanied by pain. This makes one wonder if the painless Braxton-Hicks are further proof of the mind-body connection-- the mind knows the body is not ready for labor, so no pain impulse is emitted?

**Lightening:** Several weeks before actual labor begins, the baby "drops" into the lower pelvic area. This is called "lightening." This is usually accompanied by mixed reactions on the part of the mother. It does, indeed, relieve that cramped feeling under the rib cage, and breathing is much easier; however, it also brings about much more pressure on the lower pelvis, and walking becomes a whole new experience. In spite of adjustments that you will have to make for this new position of your baby, you will find, like most other mothers, that your excitement begins to build.

From day to day you'll experience more of the Braxton-Hicks-type sensations. As you move and walk, you may even feel a sharp jolt as the pelvic area begins to make room for the baby's journey. Your body is telling you that it, too, is "ready."

Occasionally, a slight leaking of amniotic fluid is experienced. Amniotic fluid is that clear liquid within an inner membrane that supports your baby. While it may be a bit disconcerting and sometimes embarrassing when you experience this kind of leaking, there is no real danger. Nature promptly manufactures more fluid to replace that lost through leakage. Should this become more than slight spotting or leaking or if you detect an odor or discoloration, you should inform your medical caregiver immediately.

*"Express your feelings and ask questions that remain unresolved."*
*Gayle Peterson*
*An Easier Childbirth*

# *Looking at your "Due Date"*

What if your EDD (Estimated Due Date) arrives and labor doesn't start? A whole new set of feelings can spring up. Emotionally and physically you feel ready "to go"--to birth your baby--but it isn't happening. If you take your due date as gospel and you're not prepared for a possible delay, these days of anticipation can take a toll on you. You may find that anxious, well-meaning family members begin to call regularly to check; your doctor will begin to take a more watchful eye; fears concerning the baby's well being can creep in; and each day can start and end with a feeling of disappointment.

Perhaps you'll hear many stories from your friends who chose to be induced when the baby was "overdue." You may even be tempted to accept the subtle suggestions that you don't really need to wait any longer or that, ". . .you can be home for the holiday or the weekend." The important thing for you to do is continue to relax.

Before overreacting to outside pressures, remember that the estimated due date is just that--an estimation. Some suggest that it would be more realistic to refer to a birth month or to a segment of the month-- "Sometime during the first part of October. . ." or "Toward the end of September. . . ."

It's interesting to note that the number of babies who arrive on their due date is only around 5%; so, if your birthing is not "on time", relax. You will be among the 95% of parents whose babies are born in advance of the EDD or sometime after the appointed date. The gestation period for 95% of normal babies lies within a very broad range of 265 to 300 days from the first day of the mother's last period. The average, taken from those figures is the 282 days usually used to estimate the due date.

There are several reasons why your due date is only an estimation. To begin with, the selected date is usually calculated by recalling the date of the first day of your last menstrual period (which may not be accurate); counting back three months from that date; and then adding seven days. However, recent studies suggest that for first-time moms, 15 days should be added, and 10 days for other moms. Full term is considered ten lunar months of twenty-eight days each.

There are several factors that can skew this estimate: a) Actual calendar months differ in length; b) Menstrual cycles differ in the number of days between periods and in the duration of a period; c) The length of gestation can vary; d) Detection of a heartbeat or fetal movement may seem to support the timely development of the fetus at a given point; but it must be remembered that just as children differ in their development, so, too, do babies in the uterus.

For your baby's sake, you will want to resist the temptation to bring medical intervention to your pregnancy when you pass your due date. This should occur only when a medical necessity exists for you or your baby. The artificial induction of labor for a baby whose term has been mistakenly calculated could result in birthing a premature baby. It can also mean further medical procedures if your cervix is not "ripe" and ready for birthing. Neither your body nor your baby understands this arbitrary timetable, so take the due date in stride and let Mother Nature and your baby play out their intended roles in their own time. It is the safest and most natural way.

# *Avoiding Artificial Induction*

In the event that you have gone beyond your estimated due date and there is no medical urgency calling for the immediate start of labor, you still have the option of employing natural induction techniques to initiate uterine surges.

Before resorting to medication, drugs, or artificial rupture of the membrane, you need to consider what possible risks might be involved. Natural techniques are safer for you and your baby, for they allow you a comfortable start of labor and ease the impact of labor upon your baby.

If your membrane releases early and true labor does not start shortly after, you may begin hearing of the dangers of infection, followed by the suggestion that labor be induced soon. You may be asked to come into the hospital so that antibiotics can be administered to prevent infection and so that you can be monitored.

While infection is a possibility, the incidence of infection is very small. The release of the membrane in itself does not need to lead to your being rushed into artificial induction. Some doctors will want to see labor initiated if it has not started on its own after six hours. The more sensitive, mother-oriented doctors are less aggressive, some willing to wait as long as 36 hours or more if the baby's heart rate is strong and the mother also appears to be strong and in good spirits.

Pitocin, or synthetic oxytocin, is most commonly used to start labor or strengthen a slowed labor. Requesting or agreeing to the introduction of Pitocin when there is no medical need results in a trade-off that can start you on a very slippery slope. The force of Pitocin can lead to longer, closer, and more intense contractions of the uterus, subjecting you and your baby to a tumultuous birth experience, as well as decreasing the supply of oxygen going to the uterus and, therefore, to the baby. Synthetic oxytocin is <u>not</u> the same, kinder hormone that Mother Nature provides, and it can rob you of the satisfying birth you have planned.

When Pitocin is used to induce labor, it is not uncommon that it is followed by an epidural anesthesia to quell its effects. Epidurals, however, also have a trade-off. They can cause reduced muscle tone and can result in a prolonged labor. Under the numbing effects of the epidural, the mother is not aware of her surges and cannot efficiently assist in working with them. Since labor is prolonged, it can then become necessary to administer more Pitocin and so on.

The arbitrary use of Pitocin, as well as its safety, is still questionable. By the suggestion of drug manufacturers, Pitocin is not recommended for the elective inducement of labor (Physician's Desk Reference, 1994.) The American Society of Hospital Pharmacists also advise against Pitocin-induced labor except in the case of medical necessity.

If it should become medically necessary to induce labor with Pitocin, it should be administered in minimal doses and discontinued once your body takes over and labor has picked up.

Artificial rupturing of the membrane is also a means of initiating labor. While some women find no difference in the strength of the surge, others report that they experienced surges that were much more intense after the membrane had been ruptured. Maintaining your membrane in tact can ease the impact of your surges. When the membrane is left in tact, the baby's head is cushioned as it makes its way down.

# *When Labor Needs Some Help*

While simply going beyond your due date is not by itself cause to bring about medical intervention, there are some medically risky situations that require evaluation by your caregiver to protect the safety of you and/or your baby. Such instances include:

- A <u>prolonged</u> period of time from the release of the membrane without the natural start of labor
- The mother's having a highly elevated blood pressure
- A deficiency in the functioning of the placenta
- Fetal distress
- The presence of a significant amount of meconium in the amniotic fluid
- The physical health of the mother or baby is at risk
- Excessive vaginal bleeding
- Evidence of a prolapsed cord
- Indication of infection or fever

## INDUCING LABOR NATURALLY

Absent these factors, your relaxed attitude can work wonders in bringing about a natural start to your labor along with these other safe, labor-inducing techniques that you can use naturally and easily:

1. **Hot and spicy foods--Mexican or Italian**. The "beer and pizza" startup has more than occasional success. Enjoy a glass of wine with your spicy meal. Since you are at the end of your pregnancy, your baby's

development will not be at risk at this point--<u>one</u> glass of a mild alcoholic beverage may provide you with just the relaxation you need.

2. **Love-making (hugs before drugs)**. Kissing, hugging, fondling, and gentle finger or oral nipple or clitoral stimulation triggers the hormonal connection between the breast and vagina, producing the natural oxytocin that can start uterine surges. If the stimulation of one nipple is not sufficient to start surges, try stimulation of both nipples simultaneously. Prolonged or vigorous nipple stimulation is not advised, as it can have an adverse effect on your baby by creating hyperstimulation.

3. **Sex**. If your membrane has not released, have sex. The male semen contains prostaglandin, a hormone that helps to soften the cervix. Our practitioners in the Virgin Islands point out that Nature has, indeed, a wonderful plan. That which puts the baby into the uterus can nicely assist in helping to bring it out.

4. **Visualization**. While your nipple or clitoris is being stimulated, use the rosebud visualization, focusing on the rosebud's slowly unfolding and opening. Gently direct your breath down into the vaginal region while visualizing.

5. **Tea**. Drink red raspberry leaf tea or regular tea with honey. (Check with your local health/natural food store owner or herbalist for other suggestions).

6. **Walk**. Walk, walk, and then walk some more.

7. **Bath**. If rupture of membrane (ROM) has not occurred, take a medium-hot bath. It helps if you or your partner scoop the water over your nipples and your abdomen.

8. **Fear release**. Have your birth companion take you through a fear-release session similar to the one practiced in class so that you can search your thoughts to see if there are any lingering fears, emotions, or unresolved issues that you need to release. Locked-up emotions can make you feel uptight, and cause your body to produce inhibiting catecholamine. Your tension can translate into a tense cervix, preventing the flow of your natural relaxants. If you feel you need professional help, call your HypnoBirthing instructor for an individual fear-release session or ask for a referral to a hypnotherapist. It works wonders.

9. **Acupressure**. An apt acupressurist can facilitate the natural onset of labor almost immediately and yet afford you the time to make whatever preparations you need. Victoria and John W., members of one of my classes, were considerably beyond their EDD. They had tried all of the natural means they had learned in class, but with no success. Determined to exhaust all avenues before agreeing to Pitocin, they decided to approach an acupressurist. Victoria made an appointment, had the therapy, and was in labor before they left the practitioner's office. She gave birth to her baby that evening in what they both describe as an incredibly wonderful experience. If you are inclined, you can use your own skills and follow the instructions and illustrations available in many health books that cover pressure points or reflexology. **Do not apply pressure to these points other than at a time when you are ready to initiate labor.**

10. **Acupuncture/auricular therapy**. Like acupressure, there are points that an acupuncturist or an auricular therapist is able to activate for the easy and effective induction of labor. These are relatively easy procedures and offer a much smoother entry into labor. Like the acupressure points, **it is important that these points not be stimulated during pregnancy except for the purpose of induction when labor is slow to start or during a labor that has slowed.**

11.     **Primrose oil**. Primrose oil capsules can assist in naturally ripening the cervix. Prick one end of two capsules with a pin and allow the contents of the capsules to melt in your vagina daily until labor starts. Because you will be resting during the night, it's a good idea to insert the oil at bedtime. Primrose oil is an excellent supplement to take on a regular basis throughout your pregnancy and even beyond..

12.     **Cleanse the bowel**. Often the pulsating effect of emptying the bowel can stimulate the production of prostaglandin, that hormonelike substance that thins the cervix.

      a.    A gentle, disposable enema unit is easily obtained from a drug store or the pharmaceutical section of your supermarket or department store. This is the gentler of the two cleansing methods, and quite effective.

      b.    Take 1/2 tablespoon of either caster oil, mineral oil, or borage and oil every half hour for three doses. (This is made more palatable if followed by an orange juice chaser). Because the oil creates a pulsating action in the bowel, it stimulates the onset of labor.

If it is determined that artificial induction by Pitocin drip is necessary, you still may request that only a minimal dose be administered and that it be withdrawn as soon as your body takes over. You will also want to ask that the Pitocin dosage not be increased without your consent. Many of our mothers report that the HypnoBirthing relaxation techniques that they mastered successfully saw them through even with a Pitocin induced labor.

# Affirmations for An Easy, Comfortable Birthing

Here are some suggested affirmations that should be listened to or read daily during the last couple of months of pregnancy. These affirmations are on the Birthing Affirmations tape that your HypnoBirthing Practitioner includes with your class materials. If you don't have the affirmations tape, or if you wish to add some of your own affirmations to those that are listed, you can have your birthing companion read them to you, or you can create your own cassette. Be sure that your affirmations are personal, positive, and brief.

## HYPNOBIRTHING AFFIRMATIONS:

I put all fear aside as I prepare for the birth of my baby.
I am relaxed and happy that my baby is finally coming to me.
I am focused on a smooth, easy birth.

I trust my body to know what it is to do.
My mind is relaxed; my body is relaxed.
I feel confident; I feel safe; I feel secure.
My muscles work in complete harmony to make birthing easier.
I feel a natural anesthesia flowing through my body.
I relax as we move quickly and easily through each stage of birth.
My cervix opens outward and allows my baby to ease down.
I fully relax and turn my birthing over to Nature.
I see my baby coming smoothly from my womb.
My baby's birth will be easy because I am so relaxed.
I breathe correctly and eliminate tension.
I feel my body gently sway with relaxation.
I turn my birthing over to my baby and my body.
I see my breath filling a magnificent balloon.
I am prepared to meet whatever turn my birthing takes.
My baby moves gently along in its journey.
Each surge of my body brings my baby closer to me.
I deepen my relaxation as I move further into labor
I am totally relaxed and at ease.
My body remains still and limp.
I meet each surge only with my breath; my body is at ease.
I release my birthing over to my body and my baby.
I bring myself into deeper relaxation.
I slowly breathe up with each surge.
I put all fear aside and welcome my baby with happiness and joy.

# *Childbirth:*
# *A Labor of Love*

## PRELUDE TO LABOR

During those months in which your baby has been developing within your womb, it has been comforted by the closeness and warmth of the wall of the membrane that softly caresses, soothes, and nestles it. Your baby has felt the gentle stimulation of the swirling waters, and it has been lulled by the subtle movement of your body. It has heard and felt the love that you offered as you talked and played together.

Birth is going to bring an abrupt ending to that safe, secure period of life within the womb. At the moment of birth, your baby will emerge from its unencumbered world into a whole new series of experiences.

What your baby feels as it makes its way into the world can be a profusion of sensory encounters that can help make the baby's transition easy or cause him to tremble, jerk, and cringe in fear. The baby startles as it takes that first breath on its own, feels air brushing across its skin, and bristles to the roughness of fabric used to rub the protective vernix from its body. The manner in which you labor and birth and the atmosphere into which your baby is born should offer the same love and care that you provided as you carried him. You can assure that your baby's initial adjustment into his or her new surroundings is made as gentle as possible by planning and directing the course and manner of the birthing so that the welcome your baby receives is, indeed, a **labor of love**.

The environment during your birthing should be filled with the same relaxed confidence that presently surrounds your pregnancy and the calm and peace that will be prevalent during the first stage of your labor. The birthing atmosphere should be free of profuse rushing, cumbersome "setting up," unnecessary medical staff, bright lights, and careless, sometimes even violent, procedures that deny your baby's essence as a human being. There should be no loud, hurried voices telling you in cheerleader style to "Push, push, push," and "You can do it!"

Today's movies and television shows portray birth as comedic or traumatic; it doesn't have to be either. The birthing environment should have the same respect and calm as a place of worship. Great or humble, the decorum and protocol surrounding the birth of each and every baby should be conducted in a manner of reverence.

## HOW THE BODY WORKS WITH YOU AND FOR YOU

From the very beginning of your pregnancy, your body has been working for you and with you in preparation for the time when your baby will be born, assuring that when the baby is ready, your body will be ready.

The ability of your own mind that allows you to take charge of your birthing--to release, relax, and to let go, to turn your birthing over to your body--is the safest, most natural, and most effective comfort measure that you will employ through your labor and birthing. The trust that you place in this ability will create for you the beautiful birthing experience that you are seeking. That trust comes from knowing the ways in which your body works for you when you release your birthing and go with the flow and rhythm of labor.

Here is a reminder of some of the ways in which your mind and body prepare for the birth of your baby, all of which buttress the belief that the birthing process is one of the miracles of nature; and as such, it is intended to go smoothly.

## EARLY CHANGES

As soon as your mind sends the message to the body that conception has taken place, your body begins to secrete hormones that slowly turn the hard, cartilaginous substance of the cervix into loose, spongy elasticity. By the time your baby is ready, the opening of your cervix is as soft as your earlobe.

When you are confident, calm, and free of anxiety, your uterus is relaxed. This gives your baby room to respond to the pull of gravity and move from its upright position, rotating at the appropriate time and moving down into proper vertex position, ready for birth.

The relaxation practice that you learn in HypnoBirthing classes conditions your mind and body to release endorphins, the body's natural tranquilizers. These helping neuropeptides will see you through labor as you apply your skill in relaxation. When endorphins are present from the very beginning of your labor, they inhibit the release of catecholamine, the stress hormone that causes muscles to tighten and constrict.

## DURING LABOR

The longitudinal fibers of the uterus, in a wavelike surge, smoothly draw the lower, circular fibers of the uterus up and out of the way of the baby's head. Your relaxation and slow breathing, maximize the effect of the surge by helping to draw those fibers up. It is during the uptake of the surge, while you are slowly breathing up with your abdominal muscles, that you use the visualization of filling a balloon. Other visualizations of the soft, blue satin ribbons being gently drawn up and back and the opening rose are effective as you slowly exhale during the surge.

Relaxation and redirected focusing help to create a time distortion; the mind diverts attention and creates a sort of amnesia.

Hormones that have been activated at the onset of labor cause the walls of the vagina to stretch and exude a lubricating substance to accommodate the baby's moving down through the passage. The pubic region softens and spreads. The birth canal becomes even and smooth without constricting bands or protruding or thickened tissue.

The much-feared passing of the baby's head through the vagina is no more awesome than any other part of labor when you realize that there is a flexible, membranous material (fontenals) surrounding the bones at the top and back of the head, allowing the bones of the baby's skull to move. The consistency of the areas between the bones is like that of a heavy canvas fabric. Here's the good news: To allow the baby's head to adjust to the shape of the birth canal and to move that head smoothly down through the passage, the moveable bones "mold" and overlap each other, reducing the circumference of the head. Once the baby is born the bones move into their normal position, creating the fontenal space that is commonly known as the "soft spot." Until the fontenals fully close, which in some cases can take over a year for the frontal area, the soft spot is protected by the thick membrane.

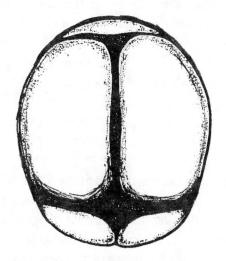

**Bone formation of baby's skull (top view)**

Pressure is a natural anesthesia. We know this when we experience the numbness that comes when we rest on a hand during sleep or when we sit on a leg for a long period of time. The perineal rim, when you have adequately softened and stretched it with massage, becomes nicely anesthetized with the pressure of the baby's head as the baby gently slips past the perineum and out of the vagina.

## *Labor Warmups*

Close to the time when you are about to have your baby, it's not at all uncommon for nature to send a preview of labor in the way of uterine surges. These contractions may even trick you into thinking that actual labor has begun. What you are experiencing is, in fact, labor; but it occurs prior to that time when the cervix begins to dilate. By sending these early surges, Nature is providing you an opportunity to rehearse your relaxation and deepening techniques. Use them to your advantage so that they don't tire you.

Unlike actual labor, the tightening sensations are erratic and do not form a pattern. The length of the surge will differ from one time to another, and there is the absence of the other signals that labor has really begun.

If you experience these tricksters, you may find that lying down or changing activity will cause them to disappear. On the other hand, they sometimes continue, settling in at five minutes apart for a day or more before real labor begins. This is the time that you want to remain in the comfort of your own home, relaxing and using some of the natural labor-inducing techniques. Those five-minute intervals often can be misleading. Resist the temptation to rush to the hospital; once you are there, you may hear the disappointing news that you have experienced little or no dilation. If you are in the hospital too early, you become an easy target for the suggestion of administering prostaglandin gel to soften the neck of the cervix, of rupturing your membrane, or starting a Pitocin drip. Well-meaning medical caregivers, unfamiliar with your relaxation techniques, begin to get concerned about your being there for any length of time without "progressing."

While labor warmups may be annoying, especially if they linger, you will want to see them for what they are, and not allow them to take on an importance so great as to overshadow the joy and exhilaration of the actual birthing that is to come.

Having said that, however, I would caution you to resist the temptation to brush off these sensations as mere early signals or just common annoyances of pregnancy. Very often women who are prepared with a relaxed attitude toward birthing and an absence of fear experience nothing more than a "real funny tightening in the pelvic area" as their first signs of well-advanced labor. Consult with your doctor or health care provider if these tightening sensations form a pattern of longer duration or shortening intervals.

## SIGNALS THAT REQUIRE YOUR ATTENTION

There are some signals that should definitely not be overlooked. You should immediately call your medical care provider if you experience any of the symptoms that are listed. Let him or her decide that it really is nothing (if, indeed, it is) or that you may have a condition that needs medical attention.

- Premature labor (three or more weeks early)
- Severe swelling of ankles, hands, face or feet
- Unusual pain in abdomen
- Excessive or continued vomiting or diarrhea
- Chills and/or fever
- Baby remaining motionless for over 12 hours (past 6-mo. point)
- Dizziness, blurred or spotty vision
- Sudden gush from the vagina of liquid that is colored or has an odor
- Bleeding from vagina or anus
- Continual, severe headaches
- Indication of infection

*"When a baby is 'ripe' and ready, true labor will begin."*

*Childbirth Without Fear*
*Grantley Dick-Read, M.D.*

# *Settling in at the Hospital*

You will probably make your trip to the hospital sometime toward the end of the early first stage of labor.

In many hospitals today you will be seen first in a triage room where your labor is assessed prior to your being officially admitted. In addition to having your vital signs taken, you will be examined to determine how your labor is progressing. Many factors are considered in triage: The length of time since membranes release; the degree to which your cervix is effaced; the number of centimeters your cervix has dilated; the pattern of your surges; and the overall conditions surrounding your labor. If your uterus has dilated between 3-4 centimeters, it is considered that you are committed to labor and a good candidate for admission.

Once you are admitted and preliminary procedures are out of the way, your birthing companion may request additional pillows and set up the tape player with your birthing music. Plan to take extra pillows from home in the event that the birthing center is fully occupied. Be sure to use pillowcases that can be clearly identified as yours so that you don't leave them behind when you are discharged or moved.

## YOUR ATTENDING NURSE COMPANION

Your nurse will become an integral part of your birthing experience and, in effect, also acts as a birth companion. The warmth, care, support, and encouragement that the companion obstetrical nurse extends is one of the most vivid recollections that a new mother carries with her as she leaves the hospital. These kindnesses remain a birth memory.

Unless your doctor or midwife is in the hospital for some reason, it is most likely that the person who will be attending you medically and keeping an eye on your progress will be your obstetrical nurse. The nurse's visits to your room and the careful monitoring of your baby's heartrate are an important part of your birthing care, not an intrusion upon it.

Most Hypnobirthing moms elect not to have continual electronic fetal monitoring (EFM) beyond the mandatory 20-minute strip that is taken upon arrival at the hospital. The EFM chart shows the fetal heart rate and the length, intensity, and distance between your surges. In the absence of any indication that your baby needs continual monitoring, his heart rate will be checked at regular intervals by fetoscope or doplar, and a gentle touch, leaving you free to move about or change position as you choose. When the monitor is used for the initial assessment, the nurse will assist you in putting on the spandex tube or the Velcro belts that will hold the paddlelike monitors onto your abdomen. Your nurse will make note of the data on your chart.

If you are birthing at home, your midwife will monitor your labor. Her assessments and your own sense of what is happening within your body will reveal to you the progress of your labor.

# *Perinatal Bonding through Labor*

Throughout birthing and labor, you, your birthing companion, and your baby will be engaged in a closeness and bonding so evident that health caregivers are almost hesitant to carry out necessary monitoring for fear of intruding on the serenity of the moment. Hospital staff are in awe as they observe you, fully calm and peaceful, responding to the touch and the voice of the birth companion as he or she sits at your side and guides you through each uterine wave. There is no doubt on the part of anyone who witnesses HypnoBirthing that the birthing companion is an integral part of this wonderful experience. It is he or she who will be the person to take the lead in assuring that the atmosphere of the birthing room is dim, calm, and serene. Your companion will be the advocate and spokesperson for you, ensuring that you experience the safe, satisfying birthing that you expect.

Your companion will usually provide any number of supportive and comforting tasks. Most helpful are the soft, whispered prompts that the companion gives as you and the baby move through each surge and wave of labor.

One of the hallmarks of a progressing labor is that your body heat begins to rise toward the end of the first stage of labor. Your companion will be there to gently wipe your forehead, neck, and shoulders with a cool and refreshing moist cloth. It's the role of the birthing companion to see that you are comfortable, with an adequate number of pillows beneath your head, back, or legs. Looking after your needs for liquids or ice chips; turning the birthing music tape; seeing that there are no unnecessary bright lights in the room; and reminding you to change position from time to time are among the welcome kindnesses that the birth companion brings to the birthing room. Touch is important and should be a constant part of the companion's involvement.

The mood of the birthing room will depend mostly on your mood and your wishes. Your birthing companion will be sensitive to and follow your lead. If you prefer to be fully conversant between surges, less attention will have to be paid to keeping birthing room activities subdued. The birth companion should be sure that trivial conversation is avoided, unless you initiate it.

If you use sleep breathing between surges, your companion will request that others keep voices soft and connect or disconnect apparatus quietly and with a minimum of flurry. As the hospital staff develops a sense of your birthing style, you will find them more than helpful. You may even find that staff members are in awe and pleased for the opportunity to be a part of your birthing.

# *The Stages of Labor*

True labor is usually defined as that period from the time you actually begin to dilate until the baby is born. Sometimes effacement and dilatation begin even prior to the onset of labor. At one of your last medical visits prior to your going into labor, your doctor may find that your cervix is beginning to efface and dilate. That does not mean you are in labor at that point, but it usually does indicate that the onset of labor is near.

Traditionally, labor is divided into three segments--First Stage, Second Stage, and Third Stage.

## THE FIRST STAGE OF LABOR

The first stage of labor is that period from the onset of regular uterine surges to the time when the cervix becomes fully dilated and the baby moves down into position for birthing.

**First stage of labor consists of four phases:**

**1. The onset of labor**--that period when labor usually makes its presence known with one or more of a variety of signals, including a sudden gush or a leaking of amniotic fluid; a "show" of bloodstained mucous; the start of uterine surges; and/or a tightening sensation across the abdomen. It is not uncommon for HypnoBirthing moms to report that a strange tightening sensation was the only indication of the onset of labor.

**2. Early first-stage labor**--that period when the uterus continues to efface and dilate to as much as 3 or 4 centimeters. Surges can range from 15 down to 4 minutes apart. If you are planning to birth in a hospital or birthing center, you will gather your bags and make your trip toward the end of this period.

**3. Mid first-stage labor**--that period when your uterus may dilate to 7 centimeters. Your surges will become closer and more effective, and labor usually moves more rapidly.

**4. Late first-stage labor**--that period when you achieve complete dilation--9+ to 10 centimeters--and your baby begins to make its journey down through the birth canal in transition.

## THE SECOND STAGE OF LABOR

The second stage of labor is when the baby moves completely down the birth canal, crowns, and is finally born. The umbilical cord is clamped and cut after it has stopped pulsating. Bonding begins.

## THE THIRD STAGE OF LABOR

The third stage of labor takes place when the placenta is expelled, bonding continues, and caregivers take whatever steps are necessary to complete medical procedures. Labor has ended.

*"Keep your sense of humor--it's a priceless gem which keeps you remembering where it's at. If you can't be a hero, you can at least be funny while being a chicken."*

Ina Mae Gaskins
Spiritual Midwifery

# *The Onset of Labor*

## WHAT IS HAPPENING

You will know that the onset of true labor has arrived when you experience uterine surges that are rhythmic--tightening and releasing in a distinct pattern. You may or may not feel your uterine surges starting. Some HypnoBirthing mothers report feeling only a tightening sensation in and around the abdomen at the onset of their labor. For many HypnoBirthing mothers, these sensations are not accompanied by discomfort; and they are not aware that their labor has actually begun.

Before or after experiencing a uterine surge, you may discover that the mucous plug has dislodged from the neck of your uterus and you have a "show" of bloodstained mucous. This show can be anything from slight pink strands to bright red, stringlike mucous.

Somewhere, at about the same time, you may experience a slow leaking or a sudden gush of clear liquid from your vagina. This is an indication that the membrane surrounding your baby has ruptured--ROM.

The start of labor may take place with all of the usual signals, or you may experience only one or two signs. The order in which they occur can differ from one woman to another and can differ with each labor for the same mother. Sometimes the rupture of the membrane (ROM), an early sign for many women, can be delayed for others until just before the baby is born.

## WHAT FEELINGS YOU MAY EXPERIENCE

You'll no doubt feel a sense of excitement and joy, mixed with relief. You will probably have a "ready to go" attitude that you will have to temper for a while. Unless you live a considerable distance from the hospital or birthing center, you will want to remain at home for as long as you can once true labor has set in. Your birthing is less apt to arouse suspicion that labor has "slowed" or that you are experiencing uterine inertia if you are not being assessed by how long you've been in labor or if you're not hooked up to an EFM (electronic fetal monitor). If your labor is not sufficiently advanced (almost 4 centimeters), you may have to return home; and this becomes a disappointment and frustration. If you remain patient and stay at home, you may avoid these emotions.

### EFFACEMENT AND DILATION

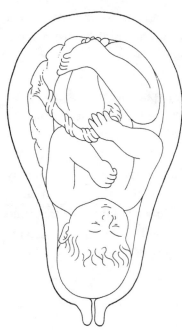 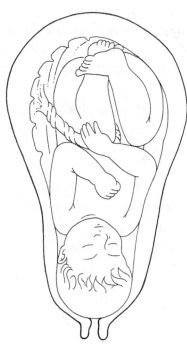

 **No dilation**                    **1 cm**

## HOW YOU MAY PARTICIPATE

The many months of conditioning and practice are now paying off. Your positive attitude and confidence will allow you to remain calm and relaxed, helping to keep your uterus relaxed.

Do anything you wish between uterine surges; but when your surges begin, use relaxation and slow breathing to increase the efficiency of each surge. In the event your membrane ruptures and you do not experience the start of uterine surges shortly after, it is a good idea to start your relaxation and slow breathing, visualizing the opening rosebud, and breathing gently down toward your vagina. This will encourage the uterus to start labor.

If you experience a delay between the time that your membrane ruptures and active labor starts, it doesn't mean that something is wrong. It simply means that it may be a while before you are be able to utilize the techniques that you've practiced so diligently. In the event that the onset of labor is delayed, you will want to refer back to the suggestions for initiating labor naturally that start on Page 114.

If your labor begins when you would normally be sleeping, capitalize on this and continue to relax and sleep. Take **light foods** for nutrition. Your body will need fuel to complete the task ahead. It will also help you avoid ravenous hunger pangs when you are in the middle of labor. Then your hunger will have to take a back seat. Be sure to drink lots of fluids and keep your bladder empty.

At your signal--usually closing your eyes and interrupting conversation-- your birthing companion will know that you are in surge and will begin to stroke your hand arm and use the cues that are on the Birth Companion's Prompt Card. It's not necessary to follow the prompts line by line. These are suggestions for the kinds of phrases that will assist you in becoming relaxed and to help you release tension. The most important prompts are that you remain limp and relaxed, that you trust your body, and that you breathe up each surge to the fullest, filling the balloon. Don't allow yourself or your birth companion to become overly caught up in the mechanics of timing and charting. You will have a sense of when the intervals between surges are becoming shorter.

If you are birthing in a hospital or a birthing center, you will want to call your medical caregiver and get ready to travel when your surges are approximately 5 to 5 1/2 minutes apart. If you have a distance to travel, you should adjust that time to accommodate your trip.

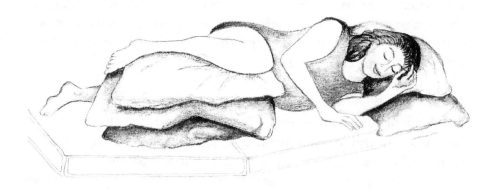

**Lateral Position During Labor**

# *Early First Stage*

## WHAT IS HAPPENING

The longitudinal fibers of the uterus continue to draw back the circular fibers so that the cervix dilates to approximately 4 to 5 centimeters. The cervix is effacing.

## WHAT SYMPTOMS YOU MAY EXPERIENCE

You will continue to experience the wave of each surge. Your abdomen will feel as though it is surging upward, tightening, and then receding back down again. These surges usually last no more than 35 to 50 seconds at this point. Keeping your body limp and relaxed allows this stage to pass with little or no discomfort. Intervals between surges can vary considerably.

## WHAT FEELINGS YOU MAY EXPERIENCE

Your mood during this early stage will usually be light and social. If you choose to, you can remain sitting or semi-sitting and conversational, or you can assume a more relaxed position. You will continue to use slow breathing during your uterine surges, working with each one to get the most out of it. If there are others in the room, you needn't feel that you have to entertain them; this can distract you from your birthing. The earlier you go within to your birthing body, the more easily your birthing will move along.

## HOW YOU MAY PARTICIPATE

Your birthing companion will guide you through each uterine wave, using the cues on the prompt card or similar words designed to lull your responses and remind you to step aside and give your birthing over to your baby and your body. You will listen to your birthing music, feel its flow, and go with that flow.

During and between surges, you will use your own favorite images of the Opening Rose, the Rainbow, the HypnoBirthing Valve, the Depthometer and Glove Anesthesia. Picturing a kaleidoscope, opening outward with its intricate colored shapes, is an effective visualization to use at this time.

When my clients in HypnoBirthing classes ask, "What should I do?" I emphatically say, "Totally relax; drink fluids and keep your bladder emptied. Other than that, do nothing!" There is nothing you can do except release and relax. Breathe up each and every surge with slow breathing so that you are working with your body; go with the ebb and flow of the tide. Give your birthing over to your body and keep out of the way. Any attempt to "do something" means that you are actually resisting the way in which the body works.

Clutching, clenching, or curling up in a fetal position--all of these motions create tension in your body that is counterproductive. You will also want to avoid getting caught up in activities and options that hospital staff will offer with kind intentions (unless those activities or options appeal to you.)

Repeatedly, I have heard mothers say that the frequent interruption of relaxation by taking walks, taking time in a jacuzzi, or spending time in a rocker, distracted them and broke their deep level of relaxation. Huffing and puffing or "blowing it away" simply saps the energy that you need to reserve for the time when you give those final one or two pushes that bring your baby into the world.

Trying to "overcome" labor can cause fatigue and discouragement. Follow the techniques that you learned in HypnoBirthing classes, and you'll find yourself fresh, alert, and fully energized when that wonderful moment of birth arrives.

*"Whenever you feel your body begin to surge, actively think "release" and "let go" of tension. There is a time for experiencing that uterine wave, flowing with it and ultimately releasing and letting go."*

*Henry Leo Bolduc*
*Self-Hypnosis - Creating Your Own Destiny*

# A Slow or Stalled Labor

One of the biggest drawbacks of having an electronic monitor in the birthing environment is that some medical caregivers tend to get overly caught up with the chart. They feel that unless there is steady progress, resulting in dilation of approximately 1 centimeter an hour, "other medical procedures" must be initiated. Often the "other procedures" are not medically necessary and serve only to "speed up" labor.

An electronic fetal monitor tracing that indicates a slow, or even stalled, labor does not automatically call for the introduction of a chemical stimulant to start up or speed up your labor. Nor do these indications necessarily mean a complicated or uncomfortable labor. If you experience a latent period when, for no obvious reason, your surges stop or the distance between the surges lengthens, it doesn't mean that your birthing has gone askew. It simply means that the uterus and your baby are resting a bit. Thoughts or discussion of "rushing" or "moving things along" or "augmenting your surges" can actually bring about the opposite effect and cause a total interruption of labor. If such a comment is made, you or your birthing companion can nicely explain that your labor is to be natural and that you are in no hurry. Nature will have its way. After experiencing the calm of a nap, you may resume an active, or even accelerated, labor.

The best way to manage a slowed or stalled labor is to meet it with patience. Once medication has been introduced, you may find that you have surrendered your choices. Before moving to other procedures, weigh the effects of chemical augmentation on you and your baby. The trade you make for a shorter time in labor may carry consequences that will turn your labor into the kind of experience that you have worked so hard to avoid.

Agreeing to or accepting the suggestion of introducing any drug into your body and your baby's body during labor can start you on a very slippery slope. Few expectant parents really take the time to explore the trade offs of deciding to use narcotics for faster birth. Rarely do they seek an opportunity to discuss the effects of labor drugs with their doctors, adopting an ostrich approach. Fear of labor can make it simpler for the pregnant mother to avoid questions concerning the risks to themselves and their babies. On the other hand, few doctors take the opportunity to explain the side effects of labor drugs with their patients. The matter becomes the medical version of "Don't ask; don't tell."

The well-respected PDR (Physicians Desk Reference) clearly states that at this time there are no adequate and well controlled studies for the use of these drugs in pregnant women. The PDR also points out that it is not known whether (these drugs) can cause fetal harm when administered to laboring women.

Even Nubain, designed to "take the edge off" labor, can suppress your efforts to work with your body's surges. An epidural, often used to quell the effects of Pitocin, also has a trade off. These drugs can cause reduced muscle tone and prolong labor. Under their numbing effects, you will be less aware of your surges and may not be able to efficiently assist in working with them. Since labor is prolonged, it can then become necessary to administer even more Pitocin, leading to continued pain relievers, and so on. During the second stage of labor, you are able to do very little in the way of helping to breathe your baby down through the birth canal unless, as often happens, the epidural is withdrawn before the second stage.

So we see a very vicious cycle--one drug initiating or increasing the contracting function of the uterus and the other reducing the impact of Pitocin but possibly slowing labor.

The same natural methods used to initiate labor can many times get a stalled labor started again. Ask for privacy so you can use natural methods--hugs before drugs. As long as your baby is healthy and you are in no danger, be willing to wait.

Occasionally, mothers find that even when they accept the suggestion of rupturing their membranes or of using a Pitocin drip, their labor does not move along more rapidly. These "remedies" can force a body into a labor that it is not ready for.

It is important for medical care providers to examine their suggestions. They should pause and consider the effects upon the mother and the baby, as well as the overall impact of the birthing experience, when they suggest intervention with drugs or early membrane rupture simply because a labor may be slow. They need to rethink Hippocrates' very old, but still relevant, dictum on avoiding, ". . .meddlesome interference." The very word obstetrics stems from the latin "obstare" meaning "to stand by." It is sometimes difficult for medical care providers, accustomed to directing and playing an active role in birthing, to adjust to waiting and "standing by" until they are needed.

Carl Jones, in his book, The Birth Partner's Handbook, quotes Dr. G. J. Kloosterman, professor of obstetrics at the University of Amsterdam, who puts it very succinctly when he says, "Childbirth in itself is a natural phenomenon and in the large majority of cases needs no interference whatsoever--only close observation, moral support, and protection against human meddling." Today, a growing number of doctors and midwives are recognizing and honoring the wishes of the mother and her birth companion and are allowing the labor to play out as Nature intended.

## COMFORT MEASURES FOR A SLOW LABOR

In addition to employing some of the suggestions in the section on inducing labor naturally, there are several ways in which you can pass time during a slow or stalled labor that actually enhance your comfort and contribute to the opening and spreading of the pelvic area. For example:

• **The Birth Ball** - The birth ball serves many purposes: It can offer you an alternative to remaining in bed during a prolonged labor; it is an excellent prop for you to support yourself by the side of your bed while your birthing companion applies Light Touch Massage; and it relaxes the pelvic muscles. Many hospitals provide birth balls for laboring mothers. Feel free to request one. They're fun.

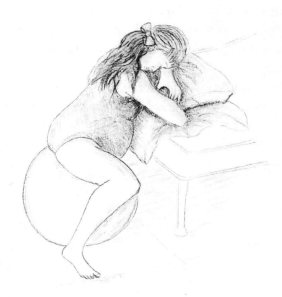

Laboring mother resting on a birth ball

- **The Tub or Jacuzzi** - Using a tub or jacuzzi provides a wonderful buoyancy that helps to eliminate that feeling of "weightiness" that sometimes accompanies birthing. Relaxing in warm water can be a comforting and soothing pastime. You will particularly enjoy resting in the tub with a warm towel covering you from your chest to your thighs. While gently scooping water over your body, your birthing companion can recite the usual prompts during your surges.

- **Shower** - A warm shower, with the water directed to your abdomen, can also be a comforting measure.

- **Humor** - The breathing produced by laughter is one of the best means of relaxing. Pack several pieces of humorous reading. Many of the "humor" sections of The Reader's Digest provide an excellent source of short, amusing stories and quips. Humor increases the production of endorphins, which, in turn, block the introduction of catecholamine, the stressor hormone that causes constriction and discomfort.

- **Nipple Stimulation** - The stimulation of one or both nipples triggers the hormonal connection between the breast and the vagina, producing your body's natural oxytocin that can enhance your uterine surges. Ask for the privacy to be able to use nipple stimulation. Your medical caregivers will be neither surprised nor embarrassed at your request.

- **Light Touch Massage** - Light Touch Massage, described in an earlier chapter, is among the exercises that you will want to familiarize yourself with. Your HypnoBirthing Practitioner will supply you with the instructions for the massage. Here again, we have a wonderful source of endorphin production.

## WHEN LABOR WEAKENS

There may come a time when all accommodation to your wishes has been extended; but, for any one of many reasons, an obvious pattern of decreased or severely weakened uterine activity forms. In such an instance, it may be determined that your birthing needs medical assistance.

Particularly, in this kind of situation, you will find that your relaxed HypnoBirthing attitude and techniques can still help you through whatever turn your birthing may take. Understanding the need for intervention and having the support of your birthing companion will help you accede to whatever preparations need to be made.

*"Prepare for a no-fault birth. . . . if you confidently participate in all the decisions made during your labor and delivery--even those that were not in your birth plan-- you are likely to look upon your birth with no blame and no regrets."*
*William & Martha Sears*
*The Birth Book*

# *Mid-to-Late First-Stage Labor*

## WHAT IS HAPPENING

Your uterine surges are closer, stronger, and more beneficial to accomplishing the goal of complete dilatation--9 to 10 centimeters. Your cervix is fully dilated by the end of this stage. The wall of the uterus is fully effaced; the baby rotates and begins its descent down and out of the uterus. The gentle, but firm, breathing down at the end of this segment helps you bypass the lengthy, difficult, and fatiguing "pushing" techniques used by other birthing methods during the second stage.

## WHAT SYMPTOMS YOU MAY EXPERIENCE

Time distortion sets in, and you begin to lose track of time. You will be aware of your uterine waves; you may or may not be aware that the surges are becoming longer and higher, lasting approximately 55 to 65 seconds. As you breathe each one up to the fullest, they become more efficient. The touch and voice of your birthing companion will ease you through each surge. As you reach the point of 6 to 7 centimeters dilated, your journey will become more encouraging, as labor from this point can move along very quickly.

You will go deeper into relaxation to an almost amnesiac state. At the end of this stage, as you become fully dilated, you will instinctively feel the need to breathe down with each surge to help the baby descend. Your breathing down will bring the baby to crowning in the second stage of labor.

## WHAT FEELINGS YOU MAY EXPERIENCE

Your mood will remain positive and calm. Your peaceful, relaxed state will turn into an almost fuzzy mood, where you will hear everything that is going on around you; but you'll not care to respond. Some mothers are able to go through this final stage of dilation in an almost dreamlike state. Nature's amnesia will lull you so that you seem to drift in and out of alertness. It becomes even easier to take yourself "out of the way," as you allow your body and baby to naturally do their work.

As time distortion clicks in, the length of the surge will be distorted, and your time consciousness will fade. Twenty minutes will, indeed, seem like five. This is Nature's way of helping you remain placid and serene.

## HOW YOU MAY PARTICIPATE

It's at about this time that you really settle into labor. Your conversant stage has passed, and you are easing into to the business of having a baby. Your deep relaxation will let you entirely turn your birthing over to your body and your baby and allow you to "step out of the way."

At the mid-to-late first stage of labor, many women adopt a lateral position. If you choose to stay on your back, be sure that the head of the bed is elevated so that you are not lying flat. Lying flat can limit the supply of oxygen to your baby. Your birthing companion should remind you to bring yourself up higher if you slip down in the bed. You will need to occasionally change position. A deepened relaxation will allow you to simply relax and let your baby and your body do what each can do best during labor. You will continue to breathe up your uterine surges until your cervix fully dilates, but it will seem almost effortless.

## EFFACEMENT AND DILATION

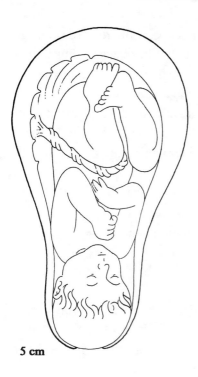

**5 cm**

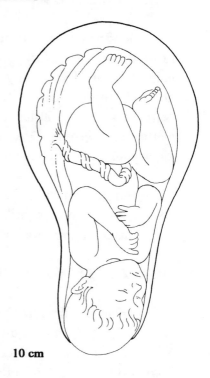

**10 cm**

Your birthing companions should take turns going for food or beverages; you should not be left alone at this stage of your labor. At this time you will welcome the touch of your companion's hand and the stroke on your shoulder, signalling you to go even deeper into relaxation.

*". . .every child is unique, every child must pass through the same stages leading from an enclosed world to the open one, from being folded in on itself to reaching outward."*
                                                                    *Frederick LeBoyer*
                                                                    *Birth Without Violence*

## Second Stage Labor

## Breathing Love--Bringing Life

### WHAT IS HAPPENING

What is happening is **Birth!** Your baby gradually descends to the rim of the perineum, and the baby's head becomes visible (crowning). Unlike other birthing methods, you will not exhaust yourself by "pushing" your baby into birthing position. You will continue to work with your surges, but with a different breathing pattern that enhances the expulsive motion of the uterus. With the head nearly or fully crowned, you are ready now to give those final few pushes that will bring the baby past the perineal rim and into the world. You touch and hold your baby on your abdomen or lower chest. When the umbilical cord stops pulsating, the cord will be cut, and you, your baby, and your birthing companion bond.

### WHAT YOU MAY EXPERIENCE

Excitement and a bit of relief; now you can **birth** your baby.

You will experience a sense of extreme fullness just above the pubic area as your baby occupies the birth canal. Your vagina will feel much like it wants to explode outward, making the wish and the urge to push stronger.

## HOW YOU CAN PARTICIPATE

Full dilation doesn't need to mean the onslaught of a sudden flurry of activity, confusion, or additional staff on the scene. It is important that you avoid any attempt to force or rush this stage. The descent of your baby can be experienced as calmly as your first stage of labor was.

It's common for hospital staff to become genuinely enthusiastic when you near completion of dilation, as they anticipate your actively "pushing" your baby down to crowning. The moves that fall into place at this time should follow the requests you expressed on your Birthing Plan. You don't want to find yourselves caught up in procedures that are different from what you have anticipated. Your birth companion will express your preference for "mother-directed" breathing down through this stage, and will assist you as you assume a position for breathing down.

Your baby's descent will be gradual. There is no need for a lengthy period of hard, violent pushing during the descent. The wave of the uterus is designed to expel, as each surge moves the baby farther down the birth path. To bear down other than when you are experiencing a surge or to give in to prompts that force you into "purple pushing" will exhaust you and press your baby against a resistent passage that is not yet receptive to his journey. Stories of exhaustive pushing that extends over hours bear out the fact that the baby will descend when he and the birth path are ready. Very recent studies suggest that forced pushing over a long period of time can be harmful to a birthing mother.

The more Nature is able to take its course, the less likely you are to need an episiotomy. A more energetic pushing will come later at near or full crowning.

The breathing that you assume now is opposite slow breathing, where you drew the surge up and worked with the upward wave. Now, instead of breathing up, you will take in a deep breath and breathe down. Your birthing companion will prompt you to direct your breath and love downward to help your baby move smoothly down to crowning. As you exhale, calmly bear down and visualize the opening of your vagina, like the petals of a rose, folding outward as your baby moves to the perineal rim.

If the move is going smoothly, you may choose to remain in a lateral position and simply breathe down until the baby's head is visible, or you may wish to adopt the Slanted "J" position, being sure to rest just above your tailbone to allow the baby plenty of room to move out.

If your baby needs help in moving down smoothly, you can assume a full- or modified-squatting or a leaping frog position to help the muscles in and around the vagina to spread and open more freely.

You should be informed of the progress of your baby's birth in a calm manner. There is a tendency for those in attendance to begin to direct this phase with loud, animated cheers. I stress that birthing is not an athletic event. Voices should not be raised. This is as much for your baby as for you. Your baby hears every sound; what he hears should not terrify him.

## WHAT YOU WILL FEEL

Most women experience second-phase labor with some impatience, but little discomfort, as they breathe down and ultimately birth. You will learn and experience the birthing process that's come to be known as "Labor." Labor at this stage takes on a slow and steady rhythm, culminating in the excitement of birth.

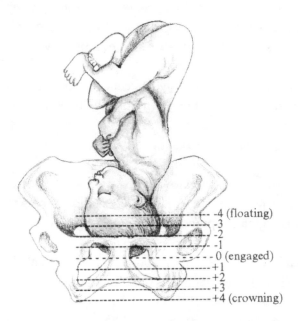

-4 (floating)
-3
-2
-1
0 (engaged)
+1
+2
+3
+4 (crowning)

## Pelvic Station

The location of the baby's head within the pelvic region is measured by what is known as Pelvic Station. Positive numbers are below the mid section; negative numbers are above the mid section. When the baby's head is said to be at zero, the head is engaged at the middle of the pelvis.

# *Positions for Second Stage Labor*

There are several positions for second-stage labor and birthing--positions that actually enhance the widening of the birth canal and shorten the second stage of labor, as well as reduce the likelyhood of an episiotomy. Unfortunately, the most common positions being used routinely are still those positions preferred by the medical caregivers--chosen for the ease of technical applications. Gradually, we are seeing more caregivers who are willing to follow the mother's lead.

I feel grateful that most of the experiences from which I've gleaned information for this writing have been in Central New Hampshire and in hospitals with staffs who are progressive in their thinking. The positions described in the following list are just a few of those usually chosen by HypnoBirthing mothers.

<u>Semi-reclining (Slanted "J") position.</u>  This very frequently used HypnoBirthing position places you reclining on a bed, <u>resting just above your tailbone</u>, with several pillows behind your head, shoulders and back. The head of the bed is elevated to a 45º angle. Usually your legs are gently spread open, supported by pillows beneath your knees. This allows the perineum to remain supple. Your birthing companion will help by giving you prompts encouraging you to follow your body's lead and to breathe love down to your baby. The position can be modified to a semi-squatting position by removing the pillows and placing your ankles against your buttocks with legs and feet wide apart and to the side. This position also widens and opens the pelvic area.

# BIRTHING POSITIONS

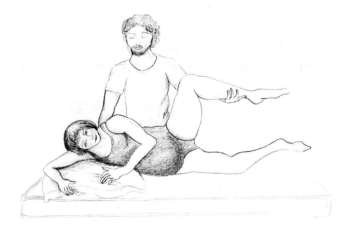

**Lateral**

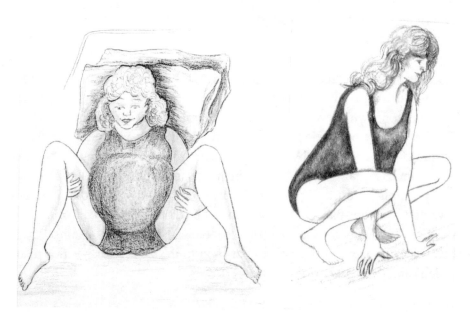

**Semi-reclining**

**Leaping Frog**

Lateral Position. This position is frequently used because of the ease with which you transition from labor into birthing. The position is the same as that used for relaxation and labor. For birthing, the leg that you rested on pillows is held up to provide clear access to your vagina.

The Leaping Frog This position came to us from our practitioners in the Virgin Islands. It is an easy form of squatting. While squatting on your toes, place your arms inside or outside of your legs and support yourself on your hands. With your legs spread to the side, this position widens the vaginal opening, utilizes the effect of gravity, shortens the birth canal, and allows you a clear view of your baby's birth. This position needs practice to strengthen the muscles beforehand, but it is worth the effort.

Hands and Knees Position The hands and knees (or all-fours) position is exactly what its name implies. Using the floor or a bed, support yourself on the palms of your hands and your knees. For variation of this position, you can bend your arms at the elbow and rest the lower part of the arm on the bed or floor. Ease your forehead or your shoulders onto your lower arms. Hospital beds can sometimes be adjusted to accommodate this position.

Toilet Sitting. Sitting on the toilet can offer the kind of spread that helps your vagina to open, utilizes gravity, and relieves you of having to support yourself on your legs. This position, of course, would have to be used prior to crowning.

Waterbirthing. The jury is still out on whether this method holds great advantage for the baby. We do know that it can relax you; and, therefore, we suggest it. But, since our mothers are quite adept at relaxation, I have found that most of them return to their rooms to use HypnoBirthing relaxation because they have become conditioned to these techniques.

# *Crowning And Birthing*

This is the first time that you "see" the results of your labor as the tip of the baby's head becomes visible. You will feel encouraged when you reach this point.

The natural pulsations of your body will slowly urge your baby forward as you direct the breathing that assists your baby to crowning.

When the top of the head is fully visible, one or two more surges are usually all that is needed to gently birth the baby's head. It is amazing how easily a head can pass through the elasticlike vulva if you remain relaxed.

The birth companion will continue to help you return to a relaxed state between surges. Birthing prompts are repeated here also. The entire pelvic area should be kept as relaxed as possible. Directing your breath toward the vagina, push the vulva outward to help open and widen the perineum.

Once the baby's head crowns, you will breathe down a little more firmly to bring the baby past the perineal rim. Tears in the skin can be avoided if there are no rushed, violent pushes. Once the perineum is fully stretched, the pressure of the baby's head will naturally provide a numbing sensation in the vaginal opening.

If you remain relaxed and if you have applied perineal massage faithfully, chances are you will not experience any burning or stinging sensation during this time. Most HypnoBirthing moms report needing only a few actual pushes to fully birth their babies.

## MAXIMIZE EACH SURGE WHEN BIRTHING YOUR BABY:

Once your baby's head becomes visible, you will begin to bear down more firmly.  This stage cannot be taken lightly if you wish to birth easily and efficiently.  You will need to follow your body's lead and work with it when you feel the onset of a surge.  Here are some helpful hints to follow when your body tells you it's surging:

- Take in a strong breath. Let the energy from your breath flow down through your body to your birth path.

- Keep your teeth together, but **not clenched**, with your tongue just touching where palate and teeth meet, mouth slightly open, bear downward to maximize your energy and open the perineum.

- You will repeat this motion several times within each surge as your body leads you through this part of breathing your baby down to crowning, bearing down for approximately ten seconds before taking in another breath.

- As you are breathing down with each exhalation, your birthing companion will help you pace yourself so that you're not letting go of the breath too soon.

- Firmly direct your breathing down through your body.  Don't let the thrust of your breath and energy escape through your mouth.

- As you get closer to crowning, gently bear down to your birth path and up in a "J" pattern--down and forward.  This helps to move your baby out and past the perineal rim.

- You may experience the sensation of needing to move your bowels, and that is exactly the region to which you need to direct the thrust of your breath, again utilizing the "J" pattern.

- These are strong, deep breaths, with the thrust of the breath going right down to your vagina. They are not shallow, panting breaths. Regardless of what position you assume, your breaths should be firm, pushing "J" breaths to assist in birthing the baby.

- Don't ride out or hang onto an individual breath beyond the point where it's working for you. Bearing down only once during a surge at this final stage will only waste your energy and cause you to lose the effectiveness of the surge. Continue to work with your body as long as it tells you that it's surging.

Your birthing companion should remind you to keep your mouth slightly open, with your lips pushed outward to help open the perineum. Totally relax the vaginal sphincter to maintain its elasticity.

Your baby is now ready to come out and must be allowed to come easily. The head births first; the vulva gradually distends without discomfort; and the baby's body emerges, often requiring only more gentle bearing down.

*"A miracle happens every day when a child is born."*

*Jan Blaustone*
*The Joy of Parenthood*

# *Bonding*

You'll not have to wait long to know whether your baby is a boy or a girl, for as soon as the baby is born, your birthing companion will announce the sex of the baby to you. You'll share this happy time together for the few seconds that it takes the medical caregivers to assess the baby's condition and suction its throat and nose if necessary.

There is no need to rush to "clean" the baby, nor to cut the cord. It is more important for the newborn to experience skin contact with both of its parents if it is at all possible. The vernix caseosa, that cheesy covering that makes your baby look like a channel swimmer, will simply be absorbed into the baby's skin.

You will experience an exhilaration beyond compare in these first few incredible moments, as you and your birthing companion touch and hold the baby, watching it begin to stretch and move, gaining a tactile sense of its new environment, one arm and one leg at a time.

Bonding during those first few, precious moments of your baby's life will provide a natural high that defies description, and the feeling that you and your companion experience will remain with you for the rest of your lives. This is when the relationship that began before your baby was born is reaffirmed with actual skin-to-skin bonding--mother, father, (or other birthing companion) embracing in loving union.

The infant is placed on your bare chest or abdomen under a warming blanket while you wait for the umbilical cord to stop pulsating. The birthing companion's hand is also placed under the warming blanket on the baby's buttocks or back so that all three of you take part in bonding simultaneously. It is at this time that a loving relationship is firmed, and this wonderful happening should not be rushed. Through your caresses and gaze and soft conversation, you validate your infant's acceptance and approval. The baby feels this love, and it nourishes feelings of security and self-worth.

HypnoBirthing practitioners who have witnessed that first gaze when the infant's eyes meet with its parent's eyes, cite this as one of the most spiritual times in their lives as birthing educators.

Like all mammals, babies are genetically and instinctively programmed to take to the breast. If you plan to breast feed, you may wish to bond with your baby in this way while the father continues to help support the baby's body with his hand or becomes involved with the cutting of the cord. Putting your child to the breast immediately has physical, as well as psychological benefits. This contact and stimulation at the breast, causes your uterus to begin to contract, helps to expel the placenta, and closes the blood vessels in the uterus. Your nurse companion will offer suggestions and assistance to help you and your baby as you experience your "first feeding."

Savor this time of bonding for as long as you wish and don't yield to the needs of hospital staff to carry out administrative details like weighing, measuring and cleaning. This is your new baby for whom you have been waiting for months. Take time to get acquainted. These moments can never be recaptured. It's important for your baby.

To be sure that your plan for bonding with your baby is realized, talk with your attending nurse sometime during your labor and remind her of your Birth Plan. Mention your wishes to have your birthing companion announce the sex of your baby and to have skin-to-skin contact with your baby, rather than have your baby wrapped in a receiving blanket. She or he will be more than happy to assist in seeing that this part of your birthing goes exactly as you wish.

*"This is a wondrous moment. You feel so unbelievably empty just afterward. One minute ago you were so tired, but this minute you feel exhilarated.*
*Susan McCutcheon*
*Natural Childbirth the Bradley Way*

# *Third Stage Labor*

## WHAT IS HAPPENING

Still at work for you, your body reacts to the euphoria you are feeling by stimulating the uterus into the third stage. Your baby takes its first breath. Medical caregivers suction the baby's mouth and throat to remove any excess mucous or fluid. The umbilical cord is cut after it stops pulsating. With one or two more surges, the placenta is born. You and your birth companion bond with your new baby.

## WHAT YOU MAY EXPERIENCE

From this point on, all who share this wonderful miracle experience a very enjoyable high. Often doctors and nurses who witness HypnoBirthing express awe at participating in the experience. An indefinable feeling of joy and pleasure sweeps in and takes over. You and your birthing companion may be oblivious to the activities of medical caregivers at this point as you experience getting acquainted with your new baby.

It is important that the cord not be cut until after it stops pulsating. When the cord is prematurely cut, it abruptly cuts off the flow of blood to the baby, depriving him of that source of oxygen. Allowing the baby to take his first breaths with the continued benefit of oxygen from the placenta eases the task of taking air into his lungs once he is outside the womb.

When the cord is clamped, your companion, if he or she chooses, may take part in cutting the cord, separating the baby from the cord and placenta.

The expulsion of the placenta should be allowed to occur naturally with just one or two pushes, as your uterus continues to surge. You may or may not be aware of these continued surges, as your placenta is birthed. These final surges help your placenta to loosen from the wall of the uterus and assist the uterus to begin to assume its normal size. Allowing your placenta to break away in this normal manner can take anywhere from 5 to 30 minutes. In the event that the placenta is not birthed within a reasonable amount of time, your medical caregiver may suggest a medical assist.

Your nurse or doctor will examine your abdomen to determine the "tone" of your uterus. If your uterus is soft, your medical caregiver may firmly massage the abdomen to help the uterus return to its normal size and substance. If you have had an episiotomy, stitches will be taken to close the tissue.

## HOW YOU MAY PARTICIPATE

During this third stage, there is really very little that you will be concerned with and participating in. Most of the activity will center around the medical staff's being sure that all medical procedures are complete. You and your birthing companion will spend your time bonding with your new baby.

Following this initial bonding, the baby may be taken to the nursery to be bathed and freshened. You will welcome this time to freshen yourself and to have your clothes and bedding changed. Very shortly the baby may be returned to you for more "get acquainted time."

An indescribable feeling of joy, excitement, and even giddiness sweeps in and takes over. Congratulations! **Your miracle is complete!**

# HypnoBirthing Stories

"Giving birth to my son was the most wonderful experience of my lifetime. My surges started almost immediately after my water broke. Once all the preliminary admission work was done at the hospital, my husband started the HypnoBirthing background music tape; and I was amazed at how easily I slipped into relaxation. My husband quietly prompted me each time I had a surge. He repeatedly gave the suggestion that natural anesthesia was relaxing me and taking away any discomfort. I could feel my body swell each time I had a surge, but I didn't feel any pain. I was conscious, but thoroughly relaxed. When it came time to push, I was actually laughing and joking. This was my first baby, and I have nothing to compare the experience with; but I know I wouldn't choose anything but HypnoBirthing for my next child."

"I am one of those people who can't stand the thought of even a slight pain. The thought of having a baby really frightened me so much that I could hardly talk about it without getting choked up. In just one class of HypnoBirthing, I became a true believer. I entered the hospital with absolutely no fear whatsoever. My faith was well placed because I went through five hours of labor and never felt a single surge."

\* \* \*

"Giving birth to my daughter was the most thrilling experience of my life. Except for the time when I was having surges, I was sitting up, talking and enjoying my husband's company. When a surge came, I easily went into a relaxed state and felt nothing but the tightness. It was wonderful to have my husband guide me through the visualizations. I was aware of the whole process and was so beautifully calm and relaxed."

\* \* \*

"I went to the hospital with all the confidence in the world. I was not at all afraid even though this was my first baby. I knew the technique and had done all the breathing practice and exercises. Just as I knew it would be, the entire experience was just great. My friends are amazed that I had such a short, painless labor. The attitude that HypnoBirthing gives you really works."

\* \* \*

"At one point I almost blew it. The woman in the next room was in terrible pain and was screaming to the rooftops. I must admit I panicked.

I wondered if, perhaps, I hadn't as yet reached that intense a point. My nurse told me that I was considerably more advanced than she. As you teach, my birthing companion gave me suggestions for deep relaxation, and all was fine. My baby was born ten minutes later."

\* \* \*

"I find myself amused at the doubt and frustrations that I experienced during your classes on relaxation. You see, I really didn't think I was accomplishing self-hypnosis. I wasn't feeling anything different. I was looking for some kind of a trancelike feeling. The things that we learned in class and from the book were just perfect. I used HypnoBirthing all the way, and my labor was nothing compared to what I experienced during my first birthing."

\* \* \*

"I had one baby with the Lamaze Method. It was an unbelievably difficult time. I was in labor for over 34 hours and suffered much of the time. When I became pregnant this time, I was looking for anything that would make it easier. My nurse midwife suggested that I try HypnoBirthing to erase some of the fear that I was feeling. I'm so happy that she did. Now, I've had one baby with HypnoBirthing; I'd say HypnoBirthing is here to stay."

\* \* \*

"There is no comparison between what I experienced with my first two births and what I experienced this time with HypnoBirthing. I would recommend HypnoBirthing to anyone. What a difference!"

"I didn't even know I was in labor. I was experiencing strong pressure in my pelvic area. I called my doctor because I thought something was wrong. When he examined me in his office an hour and a half later, he told me to go directly to the hospital and he would meet me there. I did, and my daughter was born one half hour later. I didn't even have time to call my birthing companion. I'd do HypnoBirthing again in a minute. (Maybe that's all it will take next time.)"

\* \* \*

"This is the one and only way to give birth. The midwife and all of the staff in the hospital said they had never seen a woman as strong and calm. The nurses couldn't put your book down."

\* \* \*

"Thank you for sharing HypnoBirthing. What a wonderful experience! Even though the birth took 20 hours, I was able to remain relaxed, focused, and had no discomfort throughout. My husband played an active role--stroking my arm and playing my affirmations tape. We nearly wore the tape out. I believe HypnoBirthing made all the difference."

\* \* \*

"I had doubts but went along and practiced the techniques anyway. I had assisted at two births and really didn't believe it was possible to achieve a relaxed state during labor. Once active labor started, I heard the music, heard my birth companion, and relaxed fully into that state that I didn't believe could happen. Three hours after labor started, my baby was born. I wouldn't do it any other way."

# *The Birth Plan*

The material on the pages that follow is a copy of the worksheets that your HypnoBirthing Practitioner will provide for your use in designing your birth plan. It is a good idea to complete the plan prior to your touring the facility you will use for your birthing. You may wish to discuss some of the items with the person conducting your tour.

The plan has been developed for use throughout the United States and in several foreign countries. For that reason, you will find items on the plan that may not apply to you or the facility at which you will birth. Several of the items that are listed have been adopted by most hospitals and staff long ago. However, many of the requests that are routinely honored in some geographic areas, are as yet unheard of in other areas of the country and outside of the United States. You may skip these items, mark them N/A, or extract only those that apply to your own plan.

## LETTER TO HEALTH CARE PROVIDERS:

Dear Health Care Provider:

My birthing companion and I have chosen you, our medical advisor, and you, our birthing facility staff, as the people we want to attend us when our baby is born. We have chosen the HypnoBirthing method of quiet, relaxed, natural birth. From everything we have heard from others, we truly believe that you will do your utmost to help us attain our wish for a joyous, memorable, and most satisfying natural birth.

The information that follows is a copy of our Birth Plan. My birthing companion and I have given careful consideration to each specific request in the plan, and we feel that it represents our wishes at this time. We realize that as labor ensues, we may choose to change our thinking and wish to feel free to do so. We understand that these choices presume a normal pregnancy and birth. Should a situation arise that constitutes a medical emergency, please know that you will have our complete cooperation after we have had an opportunity for an explanation of the medical need and have had sufficient time to discuss the decision between ourselves. We wish to have clear explanations of all procedures, of the progress of labor as it is assessed, and of any possible complications if they occur. In the absence of complications, we ask that the following requests be honored.

Please attach this to my prenatal record and make it available to all physicians/staff who may be attending the birth should you not be attending us. I will provide a copy for:

[ ] hospital L & D Unit         [ ] birthing clinic            [ ] my midwife

Signed:_____ Witnessed:_____

# Pre-Admission Requests

[ ]   To complete all required paperwork during a preadmission visit to eliminate interruption during relaxation for labor.

[ ]   To delay artificial induction of labor for 24 hours after the rupture of membrane if mother and baby show no signs of infection.

[ ]   To consider artificial induction only when there is a medical urgency.

[ ]   To remain at home as long as possible before going to hospital.

[ ]   To take light nourishment if early first stage is prolonged.

[ ]   OTHER REQUESTS: _____

_____

# For Hospital Admission

[ ]   To elect wheelchair assistance or to walk to my room.

[ ]   To decline routine IV prep upon admission.

[ ]   To use natural means of inducement, moving to artificial inducement only for a medical urgency.

[ ]   If necessary to initiate labor, only a minimum Pitocin drip to be used.

[ ]   Pitocin drip removed once uterus is naturally contracting.

[ ]   To return home until labor progresses further if less than 4 cm dilated or if there are no other situations that warrant admission.

[ ]   To have a private birthing room with subdued lighting and drawn drapes.

[ ]   No move from a labor room to delivery room.

[ ]   To bring a tape and player and have soft, lulling music in background.

To take enema for bowel elimination.  [ ] Yes     [ ] No
To have pubic shave "prep" around birth canal.  [ ] Yes    [ ] No
To have pubic clipping around birth canal.     [ ] Yes    [ ] No
To have the following persons present during my birthing:
[ ] husband   [ ] relative   [ ] other birthing companion
[ ] labor support person

[ ]     To have pictures or video taken.

[ ]     To have telephone calls relayed to my room.

[ ]     To have no telephone calls relayed--only messages.

[ ]     OTHER REQUESTS:  _____

_____

# During First-Stage Labor

[ ]     To have quiet room, dim lights, our own music tapes.

[ ]     To have only necessary hospital staff, please.  (We ask also that staff honor the need for quiet and refrain from any references to "pain," "hurt," "hard labor", etc.)

[ ]     To have husband/birthing companion and other labor support person present at all times.

[ ]     To be free of blood pressure cuff between readings.

[ ]     To have continuous EFM.

[ ]     To have EFM turned off after pattern is established, except for required readings.

[ ]     No EFM monitoring; intermittent fetoscope use only, please.

[ ]     No internal monitoring in the absence of fetal distress.

[ ]     No offer or suggestion of anesthetics or analgesics or labor enhancing procedures unless requested.

[ ]    Nutritional snacking if labor is prolonged.
       [ ] Fluids to sip on including juices, herbal tea, broth.
       [ ] Ice chips and popsicles.
[ ]    Freedom of choice to walk and move or not walk or move during labor.
[ ]    To change positions and assume labor positions of choice.
[ ]    Minimal number of vaginal exams--with permission--to avoid premature rupture of membranes.
[ ]    To allow labor to take its natural course without references to "moving things along," or "augmenting labor."
[ ]    To use natural oxytocin stimulation--nipple or clitoral stimulation--in the event of a stalled or slow labor, and to be accorded the uninterrupted privacy to do so.
[ ]    To be fully apprised and consulted before the introduction of any medical procedure.
[ ]    No augmentation of labor via Pitocin, amniotomy, or stripping of membranes without discussion.
[ ]    To enjoy labor tub or shower prior to ROM.
[ ]    To maintain membranes intact unless there is medical necessity to rupture.
[ ]    OTHER REQUESTS: _____

_____

# *During Birthing*

[ ]    To remain in tub for water birthing if available. (Arranged beforehand.)
[ ]    To allow natural birthing instincts to facilitate the descent of the baby, as much as possible, with mother-directed bearing down until crowning takes place.
[ ]    Use of HypnoBirthing breathing techniques--not Lamaze method.

[ ]   To birth in an atmosphere of gentle encouragement during the final pushing stage without loud "coaching." Please--calm, low, tones, free of "Lamaze-type" prompts.

[ ]   To assume a birthing position of choice that will least likely require an episiotomy.

[ ]   Use of birthing stool or bed; semi-squatting, kneeling, or leaping frog position.

[ ]   Perineal massage with oil; hot compresses to avoid episiotomy.
    [ ] Episiotomy only if necessary and only after discussion.
    [ ] Use of topical anesthetic for episiotomy.

[ ]   To decline use of suctioning device (vacuum) or forceps, unless assistance is medically necessary.

[ ]   To allow for complete birthing before suctioning baby's nose and throat.

[ ]   Videotaping of birth.

[ ]   Use of mirror to enable me to see crowning and birth.

[ ]   To have our other children present [ ]during  [ ]shortly after birth.

[ ]   OTHER REQUESTS: _____

---

# *Following Birthing*

[ ]   To have father/birth companion announce sex of baby to me.

[ ]   Immediate skin-to-skin contact, with baby placed on my stomach. No wrapping of baby. (Father/companion joins in this bonding by placing hand on baby's skin).

[ ]   Father/companion/labor support allowed to remain with me in the operating and recovery room in the event of a C-Section.

[ ]   Father will hold the baby after C-Section delivery and accompany him/her to the nursery or mother's room.

[ ]   Cord to be clamped and cut only after pulsation has ceased.
    [ ]   Father/birth companion will cut cord.

[ ]     Cord to be cut by attending health care provider after pulsation has ceased.

[ ]  Allow at least 30-40 minutes for natural placenta delivery.

[ ]     Baby brought to breast to assist placenta birth.

[ ]     Immediate massage every fifteen minutes to assist placenta birth.

[ ]     Uterine massage every fifteen minutes to assist placenta birth.

[ ]     Natural nipple stimulation to assist in placenta expulsion.

[ ]     No cord traction, manual removal, or use of Pitocin for removal of placenta unless necessary.

[ ]  OTHER REQUESTS: _____

_____

# For Baby

[ ]  To have bright lights temporarily removed at moment of birth and until baby is moved to mother's chest.

[ ]  Allow vernix to be absorbed into baby's skin; delay "cleaning or rubbing." Use of a soft cloth, not terry, when rubbing is appropriate.

[ ]  Baby to remain with me and birth companion [ ] 1/2 hr. [ ] 1 hr. [ ] 2 hrs.

[ ]  Delay use of Erythromycin or other medication for baby's eyes to allow optimal sight for bonding.

[ ]  Oral Vitamin K to be used rather than an injection.

[ ]  Please, a soft cloth or Chux pad between baby and scale.

[ ]  APGAR exam performed with one or both parents present.

[ ]  For male baby we request [ ] Circumcision  [ ] No circumcision.

[ ]  Father will stay with mother and baby throughout the hospital stay.

[ ]  To have footprints made in the baby's birth book.

[ ]  Breastfeeding several times during the first few hours of baby's life.

[ ]  Breastfeeding only.  No bottles, formula, pacifier, or artificial nipples.

# *Miscellaneous*

I would like to learn about or have demonstrated for me the following:

[ ] Proper bathing of the baby    [ ] Umbilical cord care
[ ] Taking baby's temperature    [ ] Circumcision care
[ ] Breastfeeding techniques    [ ] Using a breast pump
[ ] Formula feeding techniques    [ ] Calming the "fretful" baby
[ ] Care of nails    [ ] Diapering
[ ] Identifying signs of illness    [ ] Normal sleep patterns
[ ] Developmental ability signs    [ ] Postpartum "baby blues"

We thank you in advance for your support and kind attention to our choices. We know you join us in looking forward to a beautiful birth and celebration of this new life.

# *Testimonials*

## PARENT TESTIMONIALS

"HypnoBirthing gave me a most priceless gift--that of fearless childbirth."

"When it was time for my baby to be born, I wasn't in the least exhausted or worn out as I was from the other, more tiring breathing that I used with my first baby."

"I told myself that all I would feel is pressure--just the pressure--and it worked. Throughout the entire birthing, that's the most that I did feel, and with not a drop of anesthesia."

"My parents saw the video of my birthing, and they couldn't believe that I was even in labor."

"Nothing can describe the beauty of our birthing experience with the HypnoBirthing Program. I had two children with the other method and never dreamed that I could have as easy a labor as I did with HypnoBirthing."

"Our daughter came into this world so much easier than either of us could ever have hoped for. With Godspeed, keep up the good work of HypnoBirthing."

"When I hear women talk about how horrific their birthings were, I only wish that they had known what I know--thanks to HypnoBirthing."

"My wife's first labor was a nightmare. I was skeptical that this one could be any different. There aren't words enough to describe how beautiful this birthing was."

"Our friends laughed at us when we spoke of gentle birthing; when they saw our film, they didn't laugh anymore."

"We can see a difference in the calmness of the baby. Unlike his sisters, he is such a content baby; and he eats and sleeps so much better."

## MEDICAL TESTIMONIALS

"When Dr. Alden says HypnoBirthing is remarkable, IT'S REMARKABLE! We've practiced together for six years, and I've never seen him so excited."

OB-GYN Physician

"I'm a labor and delivery nurse. I work in this field every day, and I can hardly believe my eyes as I watch these films. It's amazing."

OB-GYN Physician

"I was at odds with my career. I even considered leaving the birthing field. Becoming a certified HypnoBirthing Practitioner opened a new frontier for me."

Certified Nurse Midwife

"I'm impressed! I'm impressed! I'm impressed!"

OB-GYN Physician

"It's beautiful! This is the way all babies should come into the world. Keep up the good work."

Labor & Delivery Nurse

"I've been delivering babies for twenty years, and I've never seen anything like this method. It's incredible."

OB-GYN Physician

"Please don't tell my wife about this method. She'll want another baby."

OB-GYN Physician

"I need an enrollment form for the HypnoBirthing classes. I'm pregnant, and I'm not going to have my baby any other way."

Labor & Delivery Nurse*

* This nurse has now had three HypnoBirthing babies.

# *Terminology for Birthing*

**ACUPRESSURE/ACUPUNCTURE**

Natural procedures used to bring about the initiation or augmentation of labor. Both are based on ancient Chinese principles of stimulating the body's natural energy flow

**AMNIOTIC FLUID**

The colorless fluid in which the baby floats in the womb before birth. It is enclosed within the placenta

**ANALGESIA**

Insensibility to pain without loss of consciousness

**ANESTHESIA**

Partial or complete loss of sensation, with or without loss of consciousness, depending on the type used

**ANTERIOR**

That which is toward the front; before; at the front

ANUS

Outlet at the end of the rectum, lying in the fold of the buttocks

BIRTH CANAL

The passageway through which the baby is born; the uterine opening and vagina

BIRTH COMPANION

Person or persons who accompany and assist the mother during labor and birth

BIRTH PLAN

A statement developed by the birthing mother and her birthing companion expressing preferences for birthing procedures

BONDING

Unique relationship that forms among the mother, her baby, and her birthing companion consisting of physical, verbal, visual, and emotional interaction during pregnancy, throughout labor, at the time of birth, and following the birth

BRAXTON HICKS

A tightening sensation in the lower pelvic area that occurs prior to the onset of labor

BREECH PRESENTATION

Abnormal position of the fetus. Buttocks, legs, shoulder, or arms come into the birth canal before the head

CAPUT

The presenting part of the baby's scalp; the crown

CATECHOLAMINE

A group of stress hormones released as a result of tension. Can have a marked effect on the muscles when tension is present. They counteract the euphoric effect of endorphins

**CENTIMETER**

> A unit of linear measure. One finger width equals approximately 2 centimeters. Full dilation is approximately 4 1/2 inches

**CERVIX**

> The lower, narrower end of the uterus, often called the "neck" of the uterus, through which the baby leaves the uterus and enters the birth path.

**CESAREAN BIRTH**

> Surgical birth that is performed by removing the baby from the womb through an incision in the abdomen

**CIRCUMCISION**

> The optional medical procedure that removes the foreskin from the penis of male babies

**COCCYX**

> The end of the vertebral column, beyond the sacrum; the tailbone

**CONTRACTION (UTERINE SURGE)**

> The muscular action through which the baby is moved down, through, and ultimately out of the uterus through a series of expelling motions

**CROWNING**

> That point in labor when the top of the baby's head is fully visible at the rim of the perineum

**CYANOSIS**

> The slightly bluish appearance of parts of the baby's skin when it is first born, usually lasting only until the baby's independent circulation throughout the body is complete

**DILATATION/DILATION**

> The gradual opening of the cervix that frees the baby to move down into the birth canal

DORSAL
> Pertaining to the back

EFFACEMENT
> The thinning of the uterine walls. Begins in late pregnancy. Cervix goes from approximately 1" to paper thin

EFFLEURAGE
> The gentle massaging with fingers or the pouring of warm water over the abdomen in rhythm with the contraction

ELECTRONIC FETAL MONITORING (EFM)
> An electronic device to monitor fetal heartbeat, and the intervals between surges and the length of time each surge lasts

ENDORPHINS
> The natural opiate produced within the body. Has the effect of a natural anesthesia

EPIDURAL
> Type of anesthesia. One of several narcotics injected around the spinal cord during labor or other types of surgery

EPISIOTOMY
> A small, straight cut made into the tissues of the perineum to facilitate easier passage of the baby through the perineal rim

EXPULSION
> The rhythmic surges of the body that move the baby out through the vagina; second stage of labor

FETUS
> The developing embryo from twelve weeks of pregnancy until birth

FETAL MONITORING
> A close check on the baby's welfare during birthing; an electrode attached to the head of the baby while in utero

**FONTENALS**
>A membranous material surrounding the bones at the top and back of the baby's head that allows the head to adjust to the shape of the birth path and move down smoothly

**FUNDUS**
>That part of the uterus that is farthest from the opening; the top

**GLOVE RELAXATION**
>A visualization technique whereby the mind creates the image of a glove that exudes natural anesthesia (endorphins) that spreads throughout the body

**HEMORRHAGE**
>Excessive bleeding

**HYPERVENTILATION**
>Condition caused by breathing that is rapid; can cause a loss of carbon dioxide in the lungs, numbness of hands and fingers, trembling, muscle cramps, and racing of the heart

**HYPNOSIS**
>An induced state of relaxation, resembling sleep, in which the client is responsive to suggestions

**HYPNOBIRTHING**
>A childbirth education program promoting natural birthing through teaching mothers self-hypnosis techniques that permit the body to work as it was created for easier, more comfortable birthing

**IMAGERY**
>The art of making images; the products of imagination

**INDUCTION**
>An artificial means of initiating labor when nature needs a boost

**INTERNAL OS**
>The opening of the cervix within the uterus

ISCHEMIA

The obstructing of the blood circulation to a part of the body

KEGEL EXERCISES

Exercises designed to strengthen the floor of the pelvis; tightening the muscles that form a figure "8" around the anus, urethra, and vagina

LABOR

The procedure through which rhythmical surges of the uterine muscles open the cervix and expel the baby, membranes and placenta

LACERATION

Tearing of skin, tissue, or muscle

LATERAL POSITION

A side-lying position used for relaxation before and during labor

LEAPING FROG

A modified squatting position used during second-stage labor

LIGHTENING

The settling of the baby into the lower abdomen in late pregnancy in preparation for birth

LOCHIA

The discharge from the birth canal during the first few weeks after delivery

LUMBAR

The area in the lower back

MECONIUM

The dark, greenish or yellow-brown bowel movement of all newborns; a sign of fetal distress if in amniotic fluid

MEMBRANES

The "bag of waters"--a sac of thin membranes in which the baby floats within the uterus during pregnancy

**MOLDING**

The overlapping of bones in the baby's head, facilitating a smooth movement down through the birth canal

**MUCOUS PLUG**

The uterine seal that prevents infection; when it breaks away, it usually signals the onset of labor with a "show" of a pink glob or strand tinged with some red blood

**MULTIPARA**

A woman giving birth to second or subsequent babies

**OCCIPITA ANTERIOR**

The normal condition during birth in which the back of the baby's head faces the front of the mother's body, its face downward

**OCCIPITA POSTERIOR**

The abnormal condition during birth in which the back of the baby's head faces the back of the mother's body, its face upward

**OXYTOCIN**

Hormonal secretion that facilitates labor by causing uterine surges

**PELVIC CAVITY**

The space within the pelvis

**PELVIC FLOOR**

The muscles and outer tissues supporting the contents of the pelvic cavity

**PELVIS**

The basin-shaped ring of bones at the bottom of the trunk of the body, supporting the spine and resting on the legs

**PERINEUM**

The opening at the external end of the vagina between the vulva and the anus

**PITOCIN**

An artificial oxytocin used to artificially induce or speed up labor.

**PLACENTA**

Organ inside the uterus that is attached to the baby by the umbilical cord. Essential during pregnancy for growth and development of the embryo and fetus--also called the afterbirth

**PODALIC VERSION**

The position of the fetus in which the feet are born first

**POSTERIOR**

Improper positioning of baby with the back of the head facing the back of the mother's body as crowning takes place

**POSTNATAL**

Occurring after the baby is born

**POSTPARTUM**

Occurring after the baby is born

**PRECIPITATE**

Describing a rapid birth, occurring unexpectedly

**PRE-ECLAMPSIA**

Combination of systems significant to pregnancy, including high blood pressure, edema, swelling, and changes in reflexes

**PREMATURE**

Describing a baby born before the normal length of pregnancy, usually weighing under 5 pounds 8 ounces

**PRENATAL**

Occurring before the baby is born

**QUICKENING**

First movements of the fetus within the uterus--usually felt between the 18th and 20th weeks of pregnancy; can be earlier

QUIET BREATHING/SLOW BREATHING

The technique of slowly breathing in and out to a designated count during a contraction

RUPTURE OF MEMBRANE (ROM)

When the bag of waters breaks or is broken

SACRUM

The triangular bone at the base of the spine--attached to the bones of the pelvis--directly above the coccyx, or tailbone

SLEEP BREATHING

The technique whereby a person is able to bring his/her body into relaxation through slow breathing--in to the count of 4; out to the count of 8

SLOW BREATHING

The special breathing that is used during a uterine surge--a long, slow intake of breath to the count of 15 to 20, while breathing up from the abdomen. The visualization is that of filling a balloon.

STATION

Distance baby's head has moved down into the pelvic region. Negative numbers are above the mid section; positive numbers are below the mid section; 0 is when the baby's head is engaged at the midpoint

SUPINE

Lying on the back with the face upward

TRANSITION

That time when the cervix is fully dilated and the fetus moves down through the birth canal; the head "crowns" at the edge of the perineum

UMBILICAL CORD

A tube-like structure connecting the baby to the placenta, 12" to 36" in length

**URETHRA**

> The canal through which urine is discharged; opening lies between the vagina and the clitoris

**UTERINE SURGE/WAVE**

> The neuromuscular motions through which the vertical uterine muscles draw the lower, circular muscles up and back

**UTERUS**

> The organ in the female pelvis in which a fetus can develop; the womb

**VAGINA**

> The passage from the cervix to the vulva, usually about 5" in length

**VERTEX**

> Presentation position where baby's head is at the lower end of the cervix

**VERNIX CASEOSA**

> The whitish, cheesy deposit covering the baby's skin at birth; word means "cheesy varnish." If left undisturbed, it is gradually absorbed into the baby's skin

**VULVA**

> The external female genitals, composed of the inner and outer folds of tissue (labia minor, labia major), clitoris, and vaginal opening

# Bibliography

Adrian, Cheri, Ph.D., and Barber, Joseph, Ph.D., *Psychological Approaches to the Management of Pain*, Brunner/Mazel Inc., New York, NY, 1982

Barstow, Ann Lewellen, *Witchcraze*, Pandora, San Francisco, CA, 1994

Birch, William, M.D., *A Doctor Discusses Pregnancy*, Budlong Press, Chicago, IL, 1988

Blaustone, Jan, *The Joy of Parenthood,* Meadowbrook, Deephaven, MN, 1993

Bolane, Eloise, *Life Unto Life*

Bolduc, Henry Leo, *Self Hypnosis--Creating Your Own Destiny,* Adventures Into Time, Independence, VA, 1996

Bradley, Robert, M.D., *Husband-Coached Childbirth*, Harper & Rowe, New York, NY, 1974

Carola, Robert; Harley, John; Noback, Charles, *Human Anatomy and Physiology*, McGraw-Hill Publishing Co., New York, NY, 1990

Carpenter, Carl, *Wholistic Pain Relief,* PKM Publishing Co., Penacook, NH, 1982

Dick-Read, Grantly, M.D., *Childbirth Without Fear,* 2nd Edition, Harper Brothers, New York, NY, 1953

Curtis, Glade B., M.D., FACOG, *Your Pregnancy Week-by-Week,* Fisher Books, Tucson, AZ

Dunham, Caroll, et al., *Mamatoto, A Celebration of Birth,* Viking Penguin, New York, NY, 1992

Ellerbe, Helen, *The Dark Side of Christian History,* Chapter 8

Ehrenreich, Barbara; English, Deirdre, *Witches, Midwives, and Nurses,* The Feminist Press, 1973

Gaskin, Ira May, *Spiritual Midwifery,* 3rd Edition, Book Publishing Co., Summertown, TN, 1990

Goodrich, Robert, *Natural Childbirth,* Prentice-Hall, Englewood Cliffs, NJ, 1955

Hoke, James, *I Would If I Could, And I Can,* Stein & Day, New York, NY, 1980

Jones, Carl, *The Birth Partner's Handbook,* Simon & Schuster, New York, NY, 1989

Jones, Carl, *Mind Over Labor,* Viking Penguin, New York, NY, 1986

Kerr, Mary Brandt, *The Joy of Pregnancy,* Golden Apple Publishers, New York, NY, 1987

Krasner, A.M., Ph.D., *The Wizard Within,* ABH Press, 1990

Kroger, William, M.D., *Childbirth with Hypnosis,* Wilshire Book Co., Hollywood, CA, Doubleday & Co., New York, NY, 1961

LaBoyer, Frederick, *Birth Without Violence,* Alfred A. Knopf, New York, NY, 1976

Lazarev, Michael, M.D., *Sonatal,* Infinite Potential, Inc., Bloomsbury, NJ, 1991

Longacre, L.D., *Client Centered Hypnosis*, Therapeutic Educational Group
    Publishing Co., Colorado, 1990

Luciano, Dorothy; Sherman, James; and Vander, Arthur, *Human
Physiology*, 5th Ed., McGraw-Hill Publishing Co., N.Y., NY McCutcheon,
Susan, *Natural Childbirth The Bradley Way*, Plume, NY,      NY, 1996

Miller, Benjamin; Keane, *Encyclopedia and Dictionary of Medicine,
    Nursing and Allied Health*, W.B. Saunders, Philadelphia, PA, 1990

Mittendorf, R., et al., *Length of Uncomplicated Human Gestation*,
    Obstetrics and Gynecology, V 75, N 6, June 1990

Northrup, Christiane, M.D., *Women's Bodies, Women's Wisdom*, Bantam
    Trade Publications

Palinsky, Constance, *Light Touch Massage*, 1995

Peterson, Gayle, Ph.D., *An Easier Childbirth*, Jeremy P. Tarcher, Inc., Los
    Angeles, CA, 1991

Sears, William, M.D.; Sears, Martha, R.N., *The Birth Book*, Little Brown,
    Boston, MA, 1994

Shanley, Laura, *Unassisted Childbirth*, 1990

Simkin, Penny, et al., *Pregnancy, Childbirth, And The Newborn*,
    Meadowbrook Press, NY, NY, 1984

Simkin, Penny, P.T., *The Birth Partner*, The Harvard Common Press,
    Boston, MA, 1989

Stone, Merlin, *When God Was Woman*

Straus, Roger, Ph.D., *Strategic Self-Hypnosis*, Prentice-Hall, Inc.,
    Englewood Cliffs, NJ, 1982

Taber, Clarence Wilber, *Taber's Cyclopedic Medical Dictionary*, FA Davis
    Co., Philadelphia, PA, 1992

Verney and Kelly, *The Secret Life of the Unborn Child*, Summit Books,
    1981

Weil, Andrew, M.D., *Spontaneous Healing*, Alfred A. Knopf, NYC, 1995

# *Booklets, Articles, Periodicals and Research*

Carnation Health Care Services, *Pregnancy in Anatomical Illustrations*, Los
    Angeles, CA, 1962
Cesarean Prevention Movement, *Things You Can Do To Avoid An
Unnecessary Cesarean*, Syracuse, NY, 1989
Division of Maternal and Child Health, *Prenatal and Postnatal Care*, Dept.
    of Health & Human Services, Rockville, MD
Gilman, Eleanor, *Turning Breech Babies With Hypnosis*, <u>American
Health</u>, November, 1995
Levine, Beth, *Labor Intensive*, <u>Woman's Day</u>, May, 1996
Mehl, Lewis, *Hypnosis and Conversion of the Breech to the Vertex
Presentation*, <u>Archives of Family Medicine</u>, Vol 3, October, 1994
Orr, Tamara B., *Controlling Pain through Hypnosis*, <u>Back Pain Magazine</u>,
    May, 1990
Reed, Donna, *Women's Spirituality, Goddess Remembered, The Burning
    Times*, National Film Board of Canada
Ross Laboratories, *Becoming a Parent*, Ross Growth and Development
Series, Columbus, OH, 1988
Tow, Jennifer, *Labor Support, Empowering Women in Birth*, <u>Spirit of
Change Magazine</u>, January 1998

# WHAT HYPNOBIRTHING CLASSES OFFER YOU:

1.  A study of the history of birthing and how historical and religious events <u>caused</u> birthing to become a much-to-be-feared process.

2.  Education in techniques that eliminate the fear that causes discomfort in labor.

3.  An air of confidence that comes from understanding how the birthing body works.

4.  An understanding of the ways in which your body and your baby naturally play their roles prior to and during birthing.

5.  Exploration of your body's natural ability to work in neuro-muscular harmony and efficiency so that each step of birthing is met with assistance rather than resistance.

6.  Instruction in the methods of relaxation and the control of slow, deep breathing to facilitate a shorter, more comfortable labor.

7.  Suggestions for creating an ideal atmosphere for prenatal, perinatal, and postnatal bonding.

8.  Instruction for your birthing companion in how to help you achieve and maintain relaxation through labor and birth.

9.  Techniques of alleviating fatigue and maintaining a positive mood throughout your labor.

10. Toning exercises to make the muscles used in birthing more flexible.

## *About the Founder of HypnoBirthing*

Marie (Mickey) Mongan is a former college dean with an active counseling practice in the Capital City of Concord, New Hampshire. Marie brings to her hypnotherapy classroom over thirty years' experience in education and counseling on the collegiate level and in the private sector.

Currently a candidate for a doctoral degree in clinical hypnotherapy, Mongan, very early in her career, received recognition when she was named one of five outstanding New Hampshire educators and granted a Ford Foundation Fellowship to Harvard University.

She is licensed by the State of New Hampshire as a counselor and holds certification as an advanced clinical hypnotherapist, a hypnoanesthesiologist, and an instructor of hypnotherapy. She holds many awards for achievement in the field of hypnotherapy and is the recipient of the 1995 National Guild of Hypnotists President's Award.

In the Spring of 1992, Mongan traveled to Moscow as an American Diplomat with the Bridges For Peace Foundation, where she taught personnel management techniques to Russian women.

She is the mother of four adult children, all born with the Dick-Read method on which HypnoBirthing is based.

Her practice includes group and individual work in a wide spectrum of therapy applications, in addition to the HypnoBirthing program that she shares with you in this book.